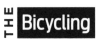

BIG BOOK of TRAINING

THE Bicycling

BIG BOOK of TRAINING

Everything You Need to Know
to Take Your Riding to the Next Level

Edited by
DANIELLE KOSECKI
Foreword by JENS VOIGT

© 2015 by Rodale Inc.

All rights reserved. No part of this publication may be reproduced or transmitted in any form or by any means, electronic or mechanical, including photocopying, recording, or any other information storage and retrieval system, without the written permission of the publisher.

Rodale books may be purchased for business or promotional use or for special sales. For information, please write to: Special Markets Department, Rodale Inc., 733 Third Avenue, New York, NY 10017.

Bicycling magazine is a registered trademark of Rodale Inc.

Printed in the United States of America

Rodale Inc. makes every effort to use acid-free ♻, recycled paper ♻.

Book design by Kara Plikaitis
Photo and illustration credits can be found on page 259.

Library of Congress Cataloging-in-Publication Data is on file with the publisher
ISBN-13: 978–1–62336–299–7 paperback

Distributed to the trade by Macmillan
2   4   6   8   10   9   7   5   3   1   paperback

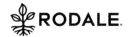

We inspire and enable people to improve their lives and the world around them.
rodalebooks.com

To all cyclists with a budding competitive streak.
Your love of the bike and willingness to challenge yourself inspires us.

Contents

FOREWORD ix

INTRODUCTION: LIMITLESS xi

PART I: PLAN

Chapter 1: Fundamentals of Fitness 3

Chapter 2: Training Components 11

Chapter 3: Physiological Testing and Training Zones 21

PART II: PREP

Chapter 4: Nutrition and Hydration 41

Chapter 5: Strength Training 67

Chapter 6: Flexibility 83

PART III: RIDE

Chapter 7: Road Skills 99

Chapter 8: Centuries 123

Chapter 9: Charity Rides and Gran Fondos 131

PART IV: COMPETE

Chapter 10: Racing 101   149

Chapter 11: Road Races   159

Chapter 12: Cyclocross   177

Chapter 13: Mountain Biking   189

PART V: TEND

Chapter 14: Your Ideal Cycling Weight 213

Chapter 15: Recovery   225

Chapter 16: Pain Management   237

FURTHER READING   **255**

ACKNOWLEDGMENTS   **259**

PHOTOGRAPHY AND ILLUSTRATION CREDITS   **261**

INDEX   **262**

ABOUT THE EDITOR   **274**

Foreword

TRAINING. WHAT DOES IT TAKE? WHAT IS REQUIRED? AND HOW CAN WE train better, smarter, and more efficiently?

Those are time-honored questions for all athletes, ones that came up quite a bit during my training journey over the years.

When I was growing up in East Germany, much of my training was based around long, low-intensity rides. As we prepared for the season each spring, we based our training around three-day blocks. For example, we would do 120 kilometers, 150 kilometers, and 180 kilometers in the first three-day block. In the next block we would do 150 kilometers, 180 kilometers, and 200 kilometers, and then, in the final block, 180 kilometers, 210 kilometers, and 240 kilometers. This program gave me lots of endurance, but I found it hard to increase my heart rate at races.

When I turned professional in 1998, my coach on the GAN team asked me, "Jens, why does a rider get dropped? It's not because he cannot do 200 kilometers at 40 kph. It's because he cannot do 450 watts for 5 minutes!" As a result, we adjusted my training to follow a more modern, sophisticated program. Suddenly I was spending fewer hours on the bike, but those hours were much more intense. And later in my career, when I started working with Bjarne Riis on the CSC team, the training became even more specific. We had intervals to build stamina. We had intervals to build maximum power. We had intervals to build speed, and we had intervals to work on our lactic acid tolerance. We were basically the first team to work in such a specific way, and for a couple of years it gave us a real edge because we simply trained smarter than other teams.

This book is designed to help athletes of all levels—not just racing pros—improve by providing a comprehensive understanding of the many dynamics involved in successful training and helping each cyclist find their perfect plan. As Danielle Kosecki has laid out in this book, you'll need a strong understanding of your body stats in order to establish your starting point. Invest in a proper ergometer so that when you measure your power output and your heart rate, you can analyze your results, or even pass them along to an expert at some point. As you modify your training, you will see your strength and your watts increasing, and with that, your speeds will increase as well. Make sure to conduct these tests in the same place, under the same conditions, as you need a constant reference point in order to produce accurate results.

It is also important to have goals. Regardless of what you're training for, goals provide focus, and all goals, be they climbing a hill faster or burning fat from your hips, are valid. Identifying your goals also needs to take into consideration the personal investment you're willing to provide.

Before you delve into the wonderful world of training, let me give you some general advice that I've picked up after 33 years of training and racing at the highest level of cycling.

1. **Don't overdo it.** This is especially true for beginners. I see it again and again—they want too much too fast and they get frustrated.

2. **Give your body enough rest.** So often people get so focused on the training that they overlook the need to recover.

3. **However, any training is better than no training.** On the occasions where you have had enough rest and recovery but lack motivation, even just an hour of training is still better than hanging out on the sofa at home watching television.

4. **Keep company.** Socialize with others. Talk about your training and try to learn what others are doing. It's always easier to train when you have a partner or a group waiting for you.

5. **Keep it in perspective:** A piece of chocolate every now and then won't kill you. As my old coach Bjarne Riis used to say, "Only a happy team is strong team!"

6. **Have fun.** This is the most important thing really. You have to like what you are doing; otherwise your efforts will be fruitless.

Jens Voigt,
former professional road bicycle racer
for UCI ProTeam Trek Factory Racing

Introduction

LIMITLESS

MY FIRST BIKE RACE DIDN'T EXACTLY GO AS PLANNED. IT WAS A COLD, wet winter morning in Central Park—less than ideal conditions, to say the least. Before the start, my teammates and I nervously waited off to the side, letting the other spandex-clad women roll their bikes to the line before tucking ourselves in behind them. We had been training hard for 3 months, but as former triathletes none of us had any idea what to expect. My oatmeal was threatening to reappear.

The race director stood in front of us and shouted our objective: three 6-mile loops ending where we were beginning: at the top of Cat Hill. Without any further fanfare, he turned the lead motos loose and blew his whistle. There was no time to be nervous now. I pushed down on my right pedal and scrambled to clip in my left while women whizzed by me. By the time I got situated I was at the back of the peloton, a place I would repeatedly find myself during the race.

At check-in that morning, an experienced rider on our men's squad had given me one piece of advice: When the pace gets tough, don't give up. Work hard to stay connected. You'll be able to rest when the pace slows back down. It always slows back down, he said.

Without that last-minute guidance, I think I would have had a much different morning. I found myself repeating his words when the pack surged up Harlem Hill and again each time someone pulled off to the side and launched an attack. This was no triathlon. Instead of riding in a strung-out line, our bikes became a mass that shifted shapes in ways I didn't yet understand. Our collective speed ebbed and flowed. One minute my quads were burning, the next I was spinning effortlessly. Each rotation of our wheels spit rain, grit, and horse crap up into each other's faces.

Three laps went by in flash. Before I knew it, we were approaching the final stretch before the Cat Hill finish. As the pace quickened, I concentrated on trying to stay in the stream of riders. When the hill kicked up and they stood to sprint, so did I. Everything was a blur until I saw, almost in slow motion, a rider's wheel fly out to the side. She went down, taking out the girl in front of me. Suddenly, I too was sliding across the wet pavement, watching the rest of the field zip by.

I know this probably seems like an odd story to tell, but it's actually one of my fondest bike memories. Yes, crashing out of my first race was pretty much a worst-case scenario, but when I think back on that day, what I remember most is standing with my coach afterward and having him put his arm consolingly around my shoulders. I think he felt bad that I had had such a terrible first experience. But I was far from sad.

I went into the race worried about getting dropped and, instead, not only hung on but had put myself in a position to contest the final sprint. I pushed my body to its limit and then found I still had more. I wasn't disappointed. I was ecstatic.

I was also hooked.

I never planned on becoming a bike racer. I'm not even sure when the idea first popped into my head. For some reason during college my boyfriend at the time bought me a mountain bike. I think he figured it would appeal to the tomboy in me, and he was right. In many ways, that dual-suspension Diamondback was a gateway drug. After tooling around aimlessly on singletrack for a couple of years, I started training for my first triathlon on it, which immediately introduced me to road biking. Eventually I saved up enough money to splurge on what I thought would be the last bike I'd ever own: a Cannondale Synapse 5. Eleven months later, I participated in that first road bike race. By the end of the year, I had added a track clinic and cyclocross race to my résumé.

If you're reading this book, it's likely that you, too, have been seduced by the bike life. Perhaps your story is like mine, and you were slowly lassoed in. Or maybe you've ridden recreationally on and off for decades and have just recently discovered the unique thrill of competition. Either way, it's clear we're not alone.

According to USA Cycling, the American governing body for all racing disciplines, the number of people participating in competitive cycling is at an all-time high. In 2013, the organization licensed 75,303 people—a 76 percent increase over 2002. However, this number fails to account for all the riders who spin their wheels in unsanctioned races, such as charity rides and gran fondos. It's no surprise that bicycling is now the second favorite outdoor activity in America (behind running), according to the 2014 Outdoor Recreation Participation Report.

Riding frequently is great, but if you want to complete your first century or tackle a time trial, you have to start riding with purpose. You have to train. This book is designed to teach you how. We've organized it in such a way that you can read it front to back or cherry-pick sections to dig into as your cycling career progresses. Here's an overview of what's inside.

Part I is all about fitness. You can be the most skilled rider in the world, but if you're not fit enough to outlast your opponents it won't matter. This section explains how to get your body in shape and how this fitness translates into on-the-bike performance. You'll learn the different ways to assess your fitness and how to use those test results to set your training zones.

Part II gets into the nitty-gritty of preparing to train and compete. Here you'll find all the nutrition and hydration recommendations, strength training exercises, and stretching exercises you'll need for day-to-day workouts and races.

Part III is where the fun begins. After a primer on road skills, these three chapters will serve as a miniguide to three types of endurance events: centuries, charity rides, and gran fondos. Besides getting a training plan for each type of event, you'll also learn which skills and techniques you should master and what to expect on event day.

Part IV takes the information in Part III up a notch. First, we'll cover racing basics and then we'll dive into these discipline-specific manuals: road racing (including one-day road races, criteriums, and time trials), cyclocross, and mountain biking. Like in Part III, you'll also get customized training plans and skills and strategy advice.

Part V addresses how to keep your body healthy year-round. It delves deeper into overtraining, explains how to optimize recovery, and tells you how to identify and reach your ideal cycling weight. Although we hope you won't need it, we've also included helpful information about caring for injuries—everything from road rash to saddle sores.

When I made the commitment to take cycling more seriously, I had so many questions. I pestered friends and teammates, read multiple books, and did endless Internet searches. The editors of *Bicycling* and I put this book together to save you that trouble. We hope it allows you to let go of any worries and doubt that you may have so that you can focus on what bike racing is all about: finding your limits and blowing past them. See you at the starting line.

PART I

PLAN

Before jumping into training, bear with us for a brief science lesson. Learning how your body builds fitness will help you understand why it's important to follow an organized training plan based on training zones. More important, when you realize that every workout is set to achieve a specific goal, it makes it much harder to rationalize skipping sessions.

CHAPTER 1

Fundamentals of Fitness

He was thinking about how it had been, when he had been in shape, and riding with the others, the pack: How his old iron bike had been a traitor some days, and his legs had laid down and died, and he had run out of wind—but how he had kept going, anyway, and how eventually—though only for a little while—it had gotten better.

—RICH BASS, AUTHOR OF THE SHORT STORY "THE WATCH"

IN ONE SENSE, HUMAN BEINGS ARE LIKE CARS: SOME ARE BUILT to go faster than others. At the elite level, the Corvettes and the Porsches are specially designed to push high speeds. Most of us are more like a Civic or a Taurus—not the world's fastest or most versatile yet capable enough to handle most rides.

While there are limits to the body you were born with, you have a much wider range of potential than you might think, says exercise physiologist Jonathan Dugas, PhD, director of clinical development at the Vitality Group, a wellness company in Chicago, and coauthor of *The Science of Sport* blog. You don't have to be blessed with the physique of Phil Gaimon or the lungs of Thor Hushovd to tap into it. Unless you've been training scientifically at a peak level for years, it's unlikely you've hit your genetic potential, Dugas says.

Your cycling abilities stem from several factors—some of which are impossible to change, while others are more responsive to training. Here's a rundown.

Muscular System

One of the ways you become a better cyclist is through muscular adaptation. In very basic terms, this is what happens: The stress of training causes microtears in your muscles. Your body then repairs the damage, which results in an inflammatory response (the swelling and tenderness you feel after a hard workout or race). This rebuilding process creates stronger muscles—but only if the body has adequate time to heal. "If you start your next ride when you're not completely recovered," says Max Testa, MD, chief medical director for Team BMC and former team doctor for the 7-Eleven and Motorola cycling teams, "your body's at a disadvantage and you'll grow more tired and gain less from each workout."

We're all born with two basic types of muscle fiber—slow twitch and fast twitch. Slow twitch fibers provide the continuous muscle contractions required for pedaling long distances. The fast twitch variety is recruited for short bursts of speed. You might think that your muscle composition overwhelmingly favors a certain type of riding, but chances are you're somewhere in the middle, Dugas says. Even at the most elite levels, athletes generally have a ratio that hovers around 60 to 40 of one type versus the other. But

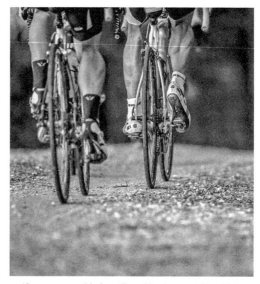

If you want to ride fast, first ride slow. Aerobic riding teaches your muscles to use oxygen more efficiently.

there's no perfect ratio. In a study of 32 elite road racers, researchers found the percentage of slow twitch fibers among the cyclists ranged from 55 percent to 85 percent. Those at the low end were among the best sprinters, and those at the highest ruled in the mountains. The key is determining your type and taking advantage of it. No amount of saddle time will alter your proportion, Dugas says, but you can train your body to use both muscle types better. Put in enough base miles, for example, and your fast twitch fibers develop more mitochondria (the structures in cells that produce power) and become more resistant to fatigue.

Power is the force applied to the pedals (leg strength) multiplied by the velocity of the pedals (leg speed). It's one physiological trait that's ruled mostly by your DNA. You need both strength and speed to develop power. In general, more muscle mass means more power, but it's not quite as simple as that. The amount of power you can produce is directly proportional to how much muscle fiber you have and how much of it you can activate at a given time. For reasons that scientists still don't entirely understand, some people are able to activate a higher proportion of their muscle fibers than others. Training can only incrementally increase this. The leg strength you develop in the gym is absolutely necessary, but it's not enough to generate power on

the bike because the exercise speed is very low (about 10 repetitions per minute). To be powerful on the bike, you must develop speed-specific leg strength by working at the desired speed with power intervals.

Aerobic System

Aerobic capacity is what it's all about for cyclists—the ability of your heart and lungs to deliver blood and oxygen to working muscles, and your muscles' ability to use these energy sources to move you down the road or trail. Your slow twitch muscle fibers rely on oxygen to turn stored carbohydrates into energy. The more oxygen your body can use, the longer and stronger you can ride without going "anaerobic," the point where your muscles start relying on fast twitch fibers to blast away at stored glycogen without oxygen, dumping muscle-searing metabolic waste, like lactic acid, into your bloodstream.

The first way cyclists typically increase their oxygen consumption is via the heart. Hours of base-building aerobic riding make your heart pump bigger and stronger, so every beat pushes more oxygen-rich blood through your body. It also creates new capillaries, tiny blood vessels that irrigate working muscles and deliver oxygen where it's needed most. Your mitochondria also multiply and enlarge. And you churn out more enzymes that help turn stored fuel into energy. These adaptations can boost the amount of oxygen your body can use by about 10 percent for each minute you ride.

The maximum amount of oxygen your body can use at full exertion (measured in cyclists in liters per minute) is called maximum VO_2. It's intimately related to stamina and is the best single indicator of fitness for people of any age. The more oxygen you can get to your working legs, the longer they'll be able to keep your aerobic (slow twitch) muscle fibers churning, and the faster and longer you'll ride before lactic acid accumulates and fatigue set in.

Genetically gifted elite male cyclists have maximum VO_2 scores in the high 70s or 80s. Top women can reach the mid 60s to 70s. According to Dugas, maximum VO_2 is modifiable. The extent to which you can expect to improve it depends partly on your genes, demonstrated by a recent study in the *Journal of Applied Physiology* that linked specific genetic markers to greater increases in maximum VO_2. Your fitness level matters, too. A cyclist with average talent who hasn't been training at a high level might see a maximum VO_2 increase of 20 to 30 percent after training, regardless of his genetic blueprint, while a naturally gifted athlete or one who starts with a high maximum VO_2 might improve only 10 percent.

Anaerobic System

The anaerobic energy system, which comes into play during sprinting, hill jamming, and other brief high-intensity work, is a key indicator of high-level fitness. Lactate, your body's buffering agent, neutralizes the acid that builds up in your legs and makes them burn during heavy exertion. The harder you turn the cranks, the faster acid accumulates. Eventually, your muscles generate more acid than you can neutralize and your searing muscles force you to ease up. The point at which you begin to accumulate acid more quickly than you can dissipate it is called your lactate threshold (also known as anaerobic threshold). In riding terms, this is the point at which you cross from comfortable aerobic riding into the red zone. It's a key performance index for people of any age, and is much more trainable than maximum VO_2.

"For the longest time, everyone focused his or her training around max heart rate," says USA Cycling expert coach Margaret Kadlick. "Now we know lactate threshold is much more important. When you raise your lactate threshold, you can produce more power at a comfortable heart rate, and that makes you a better rider and racer in every situation." With proper training (usually painful intervals), top cyclists can expect to raise their lactate threshold to more than 90 percent of maximum heart rate. Ride above about 93 percent of maximum heart rate, and you're destined to blow.

Lactic Acid Is Your Friend—Not Your Enemy

Scientists now dispute the notion that cyclists and other athletes have accepted for nearly a century—that lactic acid is a waste product of muscles overwhelmed by anaerobic energy demands. This theory is based on experiments in frog muscles done by Nobel laureate Otto Meyerhof in the 1920s. In contrast to this idea, recent studies suggest that the lactate produced by muscles helps fuel high-intensity training.

George A. Brooks, PhD, professor of integrative biology at the University of California, Berkeley, is among those challenging Meyerhof's findings. According to Brooks, lactic acid isn't a waste by-product but a kind of fuel for our muscles. He suggests that our bodies make lactic acid and break it down into lactate, which is converted by the cell's mitochondria into an important source of energy. A 2005 study from the University of New Mexico and California State University, Sacramento, confirmed this idea: "If muscle did not produce lactate . . . exercise performance would be severely impaired," wrote the authors.

About 98 percent of lactic acid is converted to fuel in the mitochondria. The remainder, called acidosis—"the hydrogen part or the proton"—is probably responsible for that familiar burning sensation. "The lactate itself is benign, good fuel," says Brooks.

The good news: This doesn't negate one of the foundations of bike training. The term "lactate threshold training" is a misnomer, as it's based on the idea of riding just below the intensity at which we thought lactic acid would overwhelm the muscles with pain, but training at that level—in short, hard repeats or steady-state intervals—does help you ride longer at harder intensity by developing more mitochondria to more efficiently process the lactate. It just needs a new name. Anyone up for a Mitochondria Ride?

60

Maximum number of minutes it takes for your body to use (or clear) lactate after you finish riding. Clear it faster by cooling down with some light spinning.

LACTIC ACID FACT AND FICTION

Fact: It's a source of energy.

Lactic acid, or lactate, is a chemical that your body produces 24/7, even while you're doing nothing, says Bruce L. Gladden, PhD, professor of kinesiology at Auburn University in Alabama. Its purpose? To feed your muscles so you can move.

Fact: It's made in different ways.

When you're spinning along comfortably, your body primarily gets energy via a slow but steady process that converts fat to fuel. But when you put the hammer down, muscles need fuel faster, so they use a speedier process that taps stored carbohydrates, called glycogen. Both methods produce lactic acid, which helps supply energy to muscles. The more carbohydrates the body uses, the more lactate accumulates in the muscles and blood.

Fiction: You can blame it for the burn.

Lactic acid is not what makes your legs threaten mutiny when you're climbing or going hard. If anything, it delays the point at which you fatigue by providing fast energy when you're pushing into the red. The burn you feel when you hit your limit is probably the result of your nervous system sensing increased acidity from the accumulated lactate, according to Gladden.

Fiction: It causes post-ride soreness.

In fact, when you ease the pace, the rate at which your body pumps out lactate slows. It doesn't pool in your legs and make them hurt. Next-day soreness is more likely the result of damage to muscle and connective tissue or plain old inflammation. "The better you are at using lactate for energy," says Gladden, "the better your exercise endurance." You can teach your body to use lactate more efficiently by putting in lots of miles. But upping your intensity will do the trick in less time. Structure your rides so you spend 10 to 20 percent of the time going hard, at an exertion level of 70 to 80 percent (or higher) of your all-out effort.

Limits You Can Push

When Dan Shelby, a certified coach and exercise physiologist at Greenville Cycling and Multisport in Greenville, South Carolina, was in college in the early 1980s, he says he considered himself "hopelessly inept" at sprinting. At a spindly 5 foot 11 and 135 pounds, he was made for going uphill. Then he started riding with the best masters field sprinter in his area. "We'd do 30 to 50 sprints a week, every town limit sign, every short climb. It was crazy, but I got faster and smarter," Shelby says. He didn't often win these contests, but he transformed himself into a competent sprinter by increasing his top-end fitness and learning to hold a faster wheel to the finish—skills that helped him earn second and third places in some races.

Shelby discovered something that's likely true for you, too: It's possible to turn yourself into a different kind of cyclist—one who excels instead of accepting limitations. It doesn't matter whether you aspire to fill a display case with trophies or simply want to enjoy the mental satisfaction of having conquered a weakness. Once you learn how to assess your skills and abilities—and how your body responds to training—you'll be well on your way down the road to reinvention.

CHAPTER 2

Training Components

You need to let your form come. Tease it. All of a sudden you'll be riding, doing the same thing you've done for days, and you think: "I'm going to go hard today." You put it in the big ring and you go, and you sustain it. Then you say, "My god, I guess I am getting fitter." That's the way it should be.

—MIKE NEEL, US ROAD RACER, CYCLING COACH, AND THREE-TIME NATIONAL TRACK CHAMPION

ALMOST EVERY CYCLIST HAS EXPERIENCED THAT FIRST BLUSH of athletic improvement—when you go a little farther, push a little harder, then come back even stronger the next time. The results can be almost dizzying. Suddenly you're losing weight, getting faster, and feeling better almost every time you ride.

Then something odd happens—you begin to experience diminishing returns. Although you're riding just as hard, your performance plateaus or even declines. What you need is a planned progression of work, rest, and more work. This should occur not just in the space of a week but over months and years. Coaches and athletes have long taken advantage of this concept, calling it *periodization*. In short, periodization is a strategic plan that allows you to gradually build fitness so you can perform at your best during certain times of the year. To do this, it depends on these four time-tested training principles:

1. **OVERLOAD AND RECOVERY:** For training to work, you must overload your body and then give it adequate recovery. Overload triggers your body's adaptation response, which causes muscles to grow stronger and provides more efficient recovery. As your body adapts, the training intensity and volume must progressively increase to achieve overload, but it's crucial to do this in small amounts to avoid overtraining or injury.

2. **INDIVIDUALITY:** Don't compare your training program and workouts to the ones your buddy's using. Training is based on your individual requirements. A program that tries to train everyone the same way won't yield positive results for everyone.

3. **SPECIFICITY:** Your program must resemble the activity you want to perform. A century

rider must progressively build a program to ride longer distances. A criterium racer must develop the explosive power necessary to respond to attacks.

4. **PROGRESSION:** Training needs to progressively advance. If you don't push yourself, you'll never get better. You must increase the number of intervals, reduce the rest between sets, increase the length of the interval, or increase the intensity.

Macrocycles

To achieve overload and recovery, periodization operates in cycles. In fact, you may have heard the terms *macrocycle* and *microcycle*. These aren't elements of the newest dieting fad—they're a crucial part of all effective training programs. Macrocycles are three distinct periods of the cycling year designed to maximize your time at peak form during the height of the season. These periods are base, build, and peak. Here's what they entail and what they're designed to achieve.

BASE

This is where your season begins. Before you do anything else, get in at least 2 months of low-intensity rides. (If you've been riding a lot and feel strong at aerobic pace, you might be able to do 1 month of base work—but be honest.) If you begin high-intensity workouts without a base, your season collapses. Think of your season as a house: Without a solid foundation for the walls and roof (hard sprints and fast climbs), everything topples. When you build endurance, eventually you can get more out of higher-intensity riding and a heavier training load. "Riders who go straight into speed work can get fast on the bike," says Hunter Allen, coauthor of *Training and Racing with a Power Meter.* "But they won't have aerobic endurance, so their fitness lasts just a few weeks before they slow down."

When you ride for 2 or more hours (or less for new riders) at a steady pace—a typical base ride—your body responds with changes that allow you to use more oxygen and burn more fat as fuel, says coach Joe Friel, author of *The Cyclist's Training Bible.* For starters, these rides build more capillaries, the tiny blood vessels that deliver oxygen-rich blood to your muscles. Your mitochondria also multiply and enlarge, and you churn out more enzymes that help turn stored fuel into energy. The result: You can ride faster and longer.

INTENSITY: Ride at 70 percent or less of maximum heart rate. *Low-Tech Translation:* You should be able to converse easily, without stopping to catch your breath, the entire time you ride.

SCHEDULE: Ride four to six times per week.

VOLUME: Start at 6 to 15 hours per week, adding 2 to 3 hours a week while building.

DURATION: Two months (two 4-week cycles).

BUILD

Now the season you're creating—remember the house image—is almost ready for walls and supports, the structures that prep you for adding the roof. Continue strengthening your base with aerobic rides, but sprinkle in slightly harder workouts that set your body up for the high-intensity work to come. Experts recommend cadence workouts because they also improve neuromuscular efficiency—they help you pedal better.

INTENSITY: Base rides at 70 percent or less of maximum heart rate and transition workouts at about 80 percent of maximum heart rate. *Low-Tech Translation:* You should be able to speak in phrases or complete sentences as you ride but should have to pause for breath between utterances.

SCHEDULE: Do transition workouts 3 days a week, with recovery rides at base pace between and at least 1 day off.

VOLUME: Start with 1-hour work sessions three times a week; increase by 10 percent weekly while building. Don't add volume to recovery rides. Keep them at around 70 percent for 1.5 to 2 hours.

DURATION: One month (one 4-week cycle).

PEAK

Here's where your power comes in. With lactate threshold workouts and weekend rides that are either actual races or hard enough to simulate racing, you develop the ability to ride faster and longer just below the point where your body cries "no more!" Power at the lactate threshold is what gives you that all-around ability to hang on in all sorts of terrain, at all sorts of speeds, and to reach deep late in a ride for a finishing burst.

INTENSITY: Keep base rides at 70 percent or less. Maintain lactate threshold rides at the heart rate at which you ride your hardest sustainable pace. To determine this, see Chapter 3. *Low-tech translation:* Talking is very uncomfortable—short phrases or words only—but possible.

SCHEDULE: On the weekends, do a lactate threshold workout or race (or simulate racing). Race-like rides are rides with no regard for heart rates; do whatever you can to stay with the group (or ahead of it). Do recovery rides at base pace on Monday and Tuesday. On Wednesday, do a lactate threshold workout limited to an hour of intensity. Thursday and Friday are the days to continue recovery while also gearing up for the weekend races or hard rides. On these 2 days, do recovery rides at base pace, with 3 to 10 minutes of lactate threshold workouts to activate those energy systems.

VOLUME: Ride 10 to 20 hours per week, depending on your weekend ride duration.

DURATION: Enjoy your season.

Rest

To maintain the foundation that you've crafted to support your riding—your base, your pace work, your group rides—you need to recover properly. A cracked foundation, worn down by too much riding and inadequate rest, can halt your progression as a cyclist. "At the end of the season, you need to fill those cracks in," says Cliff Scherb, coauthor of online coaching service TriStar Athletes. "And the best way to do that," he says with a grin, "is with chocolate and peanut butter. You need that mental switch-off, otherwise you'll never

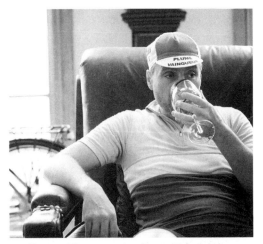

Put your bike away and grab your drink of choice. Rest is just as important as breaking a sweat.

be able to come back stronger." And he does mean off: Put the bike away, he says. Don't fret about getting fat. Accept that you're going to lose fitness, and that when you come back, you'll be as much as 70 percent off your peak. When I do come back, he tells me, "You'll appreciate going from out-of-shape guy to newly minted fast guy."

But rest isn't just for the off-season, and fatigue doesn't fly north like Canada geese when the weather turns warm. David Swain, PhD, professor of physiology at Old Dominion University, in Virginia, suggests asking yourself throughout the year, "Are you getting enough rest and recovery?" If the answer is no, "that could cause a plateau." Unless you're paid to ride, you're probably trying to slot riding in amid work and family, some weeks more successfully than others. If your life is stressful off the bike, even an easy training week can wreck you for the next one. See Chapter 15, Recovery, for more information on how to optimize rest.

Pro Tip
When training, set a goal for every ride—even if the goal is recovery.

Microcycles

Within each macrocycle are 4-week progressions called microcycles. For 3 weeks, you add volume or intensity each time you begin a new week. The fourth week is a rest week, when you drop volume and intensity to the level of the first week, or even below it. For instance, if you start your base cycle with 6 hours of riding, week two might be 7 to 8 hours of riding, week three 8 to 10 hours of riding, and week four might be 5 to 6 hours. When you begin a new 4-week block, you start at a higher level than you started the last block. For instance, in the second cycle of this base training plan, week one might begin at 7 to 8 hours of riding. One other rule: Never do two high-intensity days in a row; always rest or do a recovery ride between hard days.

Blended Periodization

Periodization works. The downside is the way periodization has traditionally been prescribed for cyclists. Because the road season runs from April through September, base building (long rides to build endurance) hits during the cold, dark months of January and February. What's more, many coaches have cyclists swear off any intensity during this period, so riders are frozen stiff and bored. "Basically, the system works for pros who can travel to warm climates to build their foundation," says Neal Henderson, founder of Boulder-based APEX Coaching and the 2009 USA National Cycling Coach of the Year. But it leaves amateur riders with day jobs out in the cold. "A better solution for these athletes is a blended periodization plan," he says. With blended periodization, you still concentrate on specific fitness goals during prescribed times of the year, but you mix it up by adding some intensity to your base building and then increase riding volume as the weather gets warmer. In the end, you'll be not only happier but probably fitter, says Richard Stern, British sports scientist, cycling coach, and founder of Professional Training Systems.

"Long rides are excellent for toughening up your behind and improving your ability to tolerate extended efforts," says Stern, "but unless you do some intensity, you really don't stimulate your cellular and cardiovascular system enough to increase your VO_2 max." In other words, taking nothing but long, slow rides can leave you a little out of shape.

On the flip side, you don't want to jam so much into January that you're flying in March and torched by June. The best thing to do in the winter is add power sprints, 5- to 10-second all-out efforts, to your riding, says Henderson. "That way you add quality to compensate for what you aren't doing in quantity, without overdoing it." Also consider substituting other aerobic activities for time on the bike. "Snow sports like Nordic skiing can be a great way to build your fitness base without burning out on the indoor trainer," says Henderson.

Annual Overview

Here's what a sample year would look like for a road racer.

MACROCYCLE: BASE

(16 weeks from late October to early February)

MICROCYCLE 1

TOTAL RIDING TIME: Ride 6 percent of your yearly hours (For example, if you set your yearly total at 250, you'll ride 15 hours in this microcycle.)

INTENSITY: Do 88 percent of your riding in zone 2 and 12 percent in zone 3 (You decide how to apportion these efforts among your rides.)

WEEK 1: Ride 23 percent of your microcycle hours (With our example of 15 hours, you'd ride 3 hours and 45 minutes this week.)

WEEK 2: Ride 26 percent of your microcycle hours

WEEK 3: Ride 29 percent of your microcycle hours

WEEK 4: Ride 22 percent of your microcycle hours

MICROCYCLE 2

TOTAL RIDING TIME: Ride 7 percent of your yearly hours (In our example, this is 17.5 hours.)

INTENSITY: Do 82 percent of your riding in zone 2 and 18 percent in zone 3 (Remember, you decide how to apportion these efforts among your rides.)

WEEK 5: Ride 23 percent of your microcycle hours (In our example, 4 hours, 1 minute.)

WEEK 6: Ride 26 percent of your microcycle hours

WEEK 7: Ride 29 percent of your microcycle hours

WEEK 8: Ride 22 percent of your microcycle hours

MICROCYCLE 3

TOTAL RIDING TIME: Ride 8 percent of your yearly hours

INTENSITY: Do 82 percent of your riding in zone 2, 12 percent in zone 3, and 6 percent in zone 4

WEEK 9: Ride 23 percent of your microcycle hours

WEEK 10: Ride 26 percent of your microcycle hours

WEEK 11: Ride 29 percent of your microcycle hours

WEEK 12: Ride 22 percent of your microcycle hours

MICROCYCLE 4

TOTAL RIDING TIME: Ride 9 percent of your yearly hours

INTENSITY: Do 76 percent of your riding in zone 2, 12 percent in zone 3, and 12 percent in zone 4

WEEK 13: Ride 23 percent of your microcycle hours

WEEK 14: Ride 26 percent of your microcycle hours

WEEK 15: Ride 29 percent of your microcycle hours

WEEK 16: Ride 22 percent of your microcycle hours

MACROCYCLE: BUILD

(16 weeks from early February to late May)

MICROCYCLE 1

TOTAL RIDING TIME: Ride 9 percent of your yearly hours

INTENSITY: Do 70 percent of your riding in zone 2, 12 percent in zone 3, 6 percent in speed work, 6 percent in hill intervals at your lactate threshold minus 5 bpm, and 6 percent in flat intervals at your lactate threshold minus 5 bpm

WEEK 17: Ride 22 percent of your microcycle hours

WEEK 18: Ride 27 percent of your microcycle hours

WEEK 19: Ride 33 percent of your microcycle hours

WEEK 20: Ride 18 percent of your microcycle hours

MICROCYCLE 2

TOTAL RIDING TIME: Ride 10 percent of your yearly hours

INTENSITY: Do 65 percent of your riding in zone 2, 6 percent in zone 3, 6 percent in speedwork, 6 percent in hill intervals at your lactate threshold minus 5 bpm, 6 percent in flat intervals at your lactate threshold minus 5 bpm, and 11 percent in racing or fast group rides

WEEK 21: Ride 22 percent of your microcycle hours

WEEK 22: Ride 27 percent of your microcycle hours

WEEK 23: Ride 33 percent of your microcycle hours

WEEK 24: Ride 18 percent of your microcycle hours

MICROCYCLE 3

TOTAL RIDING TIME: Ride 11 percent of your yearly hours

INTENSITY: Do the same as microcycle 2 but allow less recovery time between intervals

WEEK 25: Ride 22 percent of your microcycle hours

WEEK 26: Ride 27 percent of your microcycle hours

WEEK 27: Ride 33 percent of your microcycle hours

WEEK 28: Ride 18 percent of your microcycle hours

MICROCYCLE 4

TOTAL RIDING TIME: Ride 9 percent of your yearly hours

INTENSITY: Do 60 percent or your riding in zone 2, 6 percent in zone 3, 6 percent in speedwork, 6 percent in hill intervals, 6 percent in flat intervals, and 16 percent in racing or fast group rides

WEEK 29: Ride 22 percent of your microcycle hours

WEEK 30: Ride 27 percent of your microcycle hours

WEEK 31: Ride 33 percent of your microcycle hours

WEEK 32: Ride 18 percent of your microcycle hours

MACROCYCLE: PEAK

(4 weeks from late May to July 1)

TOTAL RIDING TIME: Ride 8 percent of your yearly hours

INTENSITY: Do 53 percent of your riding in zone 2, 5 percent in zone 3, 6 percent in speedwork, 12 percent in intervals with some hills and some flats, and 24 percent in racing, group rides, or adventure rides

WEEK 33: Ride 22 percent of your macrocycle hours

WEEK 34: Ride 27 percent of your macrocycle hours

WEEK 35: Ride 33 percent of your macrocycle hours

WEEK 36: Ride 18 percent of your macrocycle hours

Keep a Training Log

An essential part of any racer's arsenal is a training journal. While it's fine to use a blank notebook, these days it's easier (and frankly, more efficient) to use a web-based training platform like TrainingPeaks, Strava, or Garmin Connect.

A few things to record daily:

- **RESTING HEART RATE.** Keeping tabs on your resting heart rate—taken in the morning before you get out of bed—is one of the best ways to monitor overtraining. If your beats per minute are 10 percent higher than normal, that may be a warning that you may need to back off (see Chapter 15, Recovery, for more information).

- **WEIGHT.** Wake up, take care of business, strip down, and step on the scale—if not once a day, at least once a week.

- **MENTAL AND PHYSICAL COMMENTS.** How your body feels is another important factor to consider. On a scale of 1 to 10, record your stress, fatigue, mood, and soreness both in the morning and during workouts.

- **SLEEP.** The number of hours you sleep and the quality of that slumber both have impact on your body's ability to recovery between workouts. Staying rested also helps keep motivation high. Keep track of both the hours and quality of your sleep.

These programs allow you to not only plan and upload your workout data but also track and analyze the ebb of flow of a variety of metrics over time.

Using a modern bike computer like the ones listed below makes it simple to record the time, distance, and intensity of your rides. Uploading this data to your journal is the best way to track your progress throughout the season. To gauge how your fitness is developing, consider doing an 8- to 10-minute time trial field test every 4 to 6 weeks. Find your favorite climb or stretch of open road and track your time, distance, heart rate, and/or power over the course of an all-out effort.

Toys for Training

Whether you want to track miles, improve performance, or find new places to ride, these gadgets can help.

FOR THE NEWBIE

DEVICE: A cycling computer

FUNCTION: Tracks ride data

LOOK FOR: ANT+ or bluetooth, wireless technology that lets fitness devices communicate with each other

RECOMMENDATION: The Bontrager ANT+ Node 1.1 ($70) reads cadence, heart rate, power, and speed (with compatible ANT+ accessories) and has a customizable display

BUDGET OPTION: Planet Bike Protegé 9.0 Wireless ($55)

FOR THE FITNESS-FOCUSED RIDER

DEVICE: A computer with a heart rate monitor

FUNCTION: Tracks heartbeats per minute and calories burned and helps determine accurate training zones to reach your fitness goals

LOOK FOR: A cycling-specific unit

RECOMMENDATION: The Polar CS500+ ($320) features an oversize screen for easy one-handed navigation plus an altitude and temperature display

BUDGET OPTION: Polar CS200CAD ($190)

FOR THE LOCATION-OBSESSED RIDER

DEVICE: A GPS-enabled computer

FUNCTION: This device does everything a bike computer does, but it also tells you where you are, where you're going, and how to get there.

LOOK FOR: Downloadable maps and an easy-to-read screen

RECOMMENDATION: The Garmin Edge 810 ($500) has a touch-screen color display and turn-by-turn directions

BUDGET OPTION: Garmin Edge 500 ($200)

FOR THE SERIOUS RACER WITH CASH TO SPARE

DEVICE: A power meter

FUNCTION: Measures, in watts, the work you're generating

LOOK FOR: Either a hub unit, which is limited to the wheel on which it's installed; a crank-mounted device, which limits you to one bike; a crank arm-based meter, which is a bit easier to swap; or a pedal-based meter, which switches easily between bikes

RECOMMENDATION: PowerTap (wheel-hub units start at $790), the Quarq SRAM Red 22 (from $1,600 plus cranks), Stages Cycling (crank arms start at $700), or Garmin Vector pedals ($1,700)

BUDGET OPTION: PowerTap G3 Hub ($790)

CHAPTER 3

Physiological Testing and Training Zones

Power. Think about the word. It is what separates casual riders from the elite. You can be a precision bike handler, a wheelsucker extraordinaire, an elegant pedaler—but if you can't crank when the crunch comes, you'll be left behind.

—FRED MATHENY, CYCLIST, COACH, AND AUTHOR

MODERN BICYCLE TRAINING IS BUILT ON FOUR MEASURE-ments: heart rate, rate of perceived exertion, blood lactate level, and power output (measured in watts). When I started riding, I wore a heart rate strap and secured a running watch around my handlebars. I knew my heart rate zones but never paid attention to them. Needless to say, I quickly overtrained. If you're focused enough on racing to be reading this book, commit to using at least one of the methods above to track your training. Whether you decide to go by feel, heart rate, or power, this chapter will explain how to gauge your current fitness level and set your training zones.

Heart Rate

Compared with power, heart rate is less precise, but you can still use it to train effectively. You just need to understand what a heart rate monitor is telling you.

Power is the work you're doing; your heart rate is your body's response to that work. Heart rate data from a field test correlates strongly with power data from the same test, which means that riders without power meters can use heart rate to determine ideal intensity ranges for their workouts.

Even if you do have a power meter, you still need to monitor your heart rate. If you don't know your heart rate, you're taking power data out of context. One day, for example, you might ride a set of 15-minute intervals at 250 watts with an average heart rate of 165 beats per minute (bpm), and a perceived exertion of 7 (on a scale of 1 to 10). The next day, you might complete the same intervals at 250 watts but at an average heart rate of 160 bpm. If your perceived exertion is still 7 or 8, you should keep training. But if your perceived exertion is 9 or 10 and you feel like you're racing a time trial to produce 250 watts at 160 bpm, then you need more recovery.

Your heart rate can also tell you whether you should continue with your workout. If you've recovered from the previous day's training, your heart rate will increase as you begin an interval and you'll reach your target within 30 to 45 seconds. If your heart rate is slow to rise and stays elevated longer than normal into your recovery period, you're probably better off saving a hard session for another day.

To set your training zones based on heart rate, you'll have to calculate your lactate threshold (which experts prefer; see page 25) or determine your maximum heart rate (the highest number of beats your heart can reach in an all-out effort). The commonly used maximum heart rate formula of 220 minus age has been discredited in recent years. A 2013 study found that 211 minus 64 percent of age provides a more accurate measurement. Racers often achieve a maximum heart rate at the top of a very tough climb or at the end of a short time trial. Check your training files: The biggest number you've seen on your heart rate monitor is probably not far off if it was achieved in a competitive situation. Don't think you've pushed yourself to the max yet? Do a field test. Here's how.

After an adequate warm-up, take 30 to 40

seconds to get up to speed, then settle into the highest intensity you can maintain for 10 minutes, sprinting as hard as you can for the final 30 seconds. Cool down, then check your heart rate monitor for the highest heart rate you achieved. Repeat this test twice more (with rest days in between) to find the most accurate number.

Don't worry about your beats per minute values during short, maximal efforts: Your heart rate won't respond quickly enough to provide useful information. Just dig in and go.

Rate of Perceived Exertion

For many riders, heart rate has become training's truth serum. The theory is that using a monitor allows you to ignore how you feel and concentrate on how your body is actually performing. In other words, the numbers never lie.

Or do they? Increasingly, coaches are using a subjective gauge (in combination with heart rate) to assess gains in conditioning and prevent riders from overtraining. This yardstick of physical effort is called the Borg scale, named for its Swedish inventor Gunnar Borg, MD, PhD, professor emeritus of perception and psychophysics at Stockholm University. The original scale runs from 6 to 20. A rating of 7 is described as a "very, very light" intensity, such as when pedaling with no resistance. A rating of 17 is "very hard," or just past the anaerobic threshold (anaerobic threshold is a time-trial

pace), and 19 is "very, very hard," or close to an all-out effort. It may be easier to translate the Borg into a 1 to 10 scale (see page 24).

It's a system so simple that it seems like it can't possibly work, but it does. In a study at Southern Illinois University, runners performed a treadmill test to exhaustion. At 75 percent of maximum heart rate, they were asked to record their rate of perceived exertion. In a second test, they tried to achieve the same 75 percent intensity based on the rate of perceived exertion alone. They did so within an average of 4 bpm. Not bad. A similar study at the University of Pittsburgh that used both treadmills and cycle ergometers found that the rate of perceived exertion was even more accurate on the bike. (In this case, for achieving intensities of 50 percent and 70 percent of maximum VO_2.) Similar results have been found for everything from stair-climbing to aerobic dance.

Perceived exertion has a number of advantages. Consider, for instance, adherents to the "no pain/no gain" philosophy, who consistently ignore their perceptions and train beyond their limits. For them, the rate of perceived exertion can provide realistic feedback and prevent overtraining. It's also valuable to those unwilling (or unable) to undergo a test to find maximum heart rate. Such people try to determine their max using the wildly inaccurate formula of 220 minus age, then train at a percentage of that guesstimate. Instead, it can be more effective to train at a certain rate of perceived exertion level. (For example, an anaerobic threshold workout would occur at roughly 16 on the scale.)

So should we toss our $100 heart rate monitors and tape a Borg scale to the bar? Hardly. Not all coaches put their faith in perceived exertion, and most who do insist on combining it with heart rate, speed, and even power output to get the full picture.

If you want to incorporate perceived exertion into your training program, follow these three steps.

TAKE THE TEST

Have a copy of the 1-to-10 Borg scale nearby and note how your heart rate, particularly anaerobic threshold, corresponds to it as you increase intensity. Initially, a stationary trainer provides the most controlled environment in which to do this. I've used the Borg scale quite a bit and found that a rating of 6 to 7 consistently matches anaerobic threshold. Some testing guidelines:

- Don't allow localized pain, such as that of the quadriceps, to dominate your perception. Integrate everything you feel into one rating that includes muscular and cardiovascular demands.

- Be honest. Studies have shown that inexperienced cyclists tend to underestimate their rate of perceived exertion, perhaps out of a feeling of pride. This can lead to overtraining. Experienced riders are more realistic about the pain they feel.

- Don't compare your rate of perceived exertion ratings to those of anyone else. There is no "correct" rating.

PRACTICE

Coaches who use perceived exertion are unanimous in one thing: the value of practice. Only through repeated use will you be able to detect changes and incorporate the information into

BORG SCALE OF PERCEIVED EXERTION	
0	Rest
1	Really Easy
2	Easy
3	Moderate
4	Sort of Hard
5	Hard
6	
7	Really Hard
8	
9	Really, Really Hard
10	Maximal

your training program. "You need to keep coming back to verify perceived exertion with heart rate and pace," says Hank Lange, a triathlete and personal from Brattleboro, Vermont. "It's definitely a learned skill. As you improve at reading your body, perceived exertion becomes a better tool." For instance, Lange has his athletes record their rate of perceived exertion immediately after each workout. "This way I can see how it changes over time. Once you get it dialed in, you can start to use it very accurately to assess what's going on, and perhaps even wear the heart rate monitor less."

ACT ON THE RESULTS

Put simply, a rate of perceived exertion that is abnormally low for a given heart rate and pace indicates a gain in fitness. If this is the case, it might be time to up the ante—for instance, raise the heart rate level at which you do an interval workout. Conversely, a rate of perceived exertion that's high for a given speed or heart rate can indicate overtraining or stress. If this is the case, you might want to take a day off.

"Say you feel a perceived exertion of 6, which is your threshold level, at about 23 mph," says Rick Niles, a personal coach in Santa Rosa, California. "Then after 3 weeks of hard training, you can only go 21 mph at that rating, and your heart rate won't climb.

That's a classic overtraining symptom.

"The other thing you might see is a higher heart rate at a given perceived exertion. That's good. It means an increase in your threshold level. Overall, I've found that what people perceive exertion to be won't change. What's easiest to track is a change in performance at a given Borg reading." Don't worry—you'll get the feel of it.

Blood Lactate Level

I bet you've heard cyclists say they're "training at 90 percent of max heart rate," or some similar figure. Sounds kind of impressive, doesn't it? After all, we athletes like to do everything to the max. Although maximum heart rate is a useful benchmark for determining how intense your training should be, it isn't as effective as lactate threshold, the border between high- and low-intensity work, or roughly the effort experienced in a flat-out, 30-minute time trial. Lactate threshold is a better baseline than maximum heart rate for determining training zones because two cyclists with the same maximum heart rate may have widely varying lactate thresholds due to genetic or training differences. Sedentary people can have lactate thresholds as low as 50 percent of maximum heart rate, while elite athletes can maintain 90 to 95 percent for an hour. Once you determine your individual lactate threshold, every workout can be based on a reference point that yields safe, repeatable, focused training tailored to your fitness level at that moment. Fortunately, it isn't hard to determine your lactate threshold.

IN THE LAB

Many coaches and fitness centers offer lactate threshold tests for about $175. The test takes 30 to 40 minutes. While wearing a heart rate strap, you'll start pedaling easily on a stationary bike set up for a specific power output. Every few minutes, the resistance increases, and increases, and increases some more, until you can no longer keep going. At each increase, the technician pricks your finger for a drop of blood, which a machine then analyzes for lactate, or lactic acid, the prime marker of muscular fatigue. All the data is streamed into a desktop computer, which plots the graph of your results.

30-MINUTE TIME TRIAL

Most cyclists, however, don't have access to lab facilities to determine their lactate threshold. You can find yours with a simple 30-minute time trial that's best done outdoors on a flat road. The average heart rate you can maintain for the ride—about 10 miles—is a good working approximation of your lactate threshold.

AN INDOOR TEST AT HOME

You can also find your lactate threshold at home with this indoor test. Calculate a range from 80 to 90 percent of maximum heart rate. For instance, if your maximum heart rate is 180 bpm, 80 percent is 144 bpm and 90 percent is 162. Most cyclists' lactate threshold will be somewhere between these two numbers, depending on conditioning. Once you've estimated your lactate threshold range, perform an indoor test to find what resistance/gear keeps you in your lactate threshold range while pedaling a constant 90 rpm. (You'll need a cadence function on your bike computer, your heart rate monitor, and a friend.) Warm up well, then maintain 90 rpm in your chosen gear. Pedal for 15 minutes and have your helper jot down your heart rate each minute. If you've chosen a gear that's too high (your heart rate soars and you gasp for breath), stop, decrease gearing, and do another test on a different day using a lower gear. When you complete a test during which you are pedaling at the highest gear that allows your heart rate to stay fairly level over the 15-minute test, note that heart rate—it is very close to your lactate threshold. But remember: Don't go too easy—you are trying to find the highest heart rate you can maintain for 15 minutes (your breathing should become moderately labored).

Now—and this is important—when you've

found your final number, subtract two to five beats for your final figure. Why? Because most cyclists overestimate their lactate threshold, resulting in training ranges that are too high. Test your estimate on rides. How does this intensity feel? Can you maintain your goal heart rate? Remember that this isn't a precise science. You're merely trying to find a good number upon which to base your training. By following these steps riders can get an accurate measure of their lactate threshold within a couple of beats per minute.

Power Output

Power meters—devices that attach to your bike to measure pedal force multiplied by cadence, or how much power you're producing—are changing the entire cycling training paradigm. Using one just may make you faster than you've ever been in your life. These devices have all the features of a typical topflight handlebar-mounted computer: speed, distance, time, cadence, heart rate (all with maxes and averages), and even energy expended (so you can calculate calories burned). The key additional measurement is power, in watts, measured by sensors located at your crank, pedal, hub, bottom bracket, or chain (depending on the brand you buy).

What power devotees love best is that watts don't lie. Heart rate—the measure that most of us still base our training on—is fickle. Lack of sleep, altitude, weather, the menstrual cycle, and caffeine can speed it up or slow it down. And, most important, there's a lag time for your heart rate to respond to your effort, so you could be two-thirds of the way through an interval before your heart gives you an indication of how hard you're working.

"Heart rate monitoring became popular because it's easy, affordable, and is a number everyone can relate to," says Andrew Coggan, PhD, an internationally recognized exercise physiologist and coauthor of *Training and Racing with a Power Meter*. "But it's backassward." Your muscles' demand for energy dictates all physiological responses, including heart rate, he says. What determines that demand is the force your muscles produce, or how much power you're generating. "If you want to hit a specific heart rate, you do it by generating specific wattages, not the other way around."

ANALYZE THIS

Fancy measuring tools don't change the secret to riding faster: following a program of systematic overload and recovery. Push your muscles past the brink and allow them to rebuild, and they'll be stronger than before. But knowing your power output lets you be precise and systematic, so you reap more benefit from training. Here's a rundown of what watts help you do.

AVOID OVERTRAINING. It's easy when you know your power output, says James Herrera, owner of Performance Driven, an elite coaching program based in Colorado Springs, Colorado. "If you see a 10 percent drop in power from one interval to the next, you've achieved overload."

PREVENT SLACKING. "I look for times when I'm producing zero watts," says Mark McCormack, the first rider to hold the US national championship in cyclocross and road bicycle racing. "Now I pedal on long descents or in tailwinds. I can do the same training ride in three and a half hours that took me four without a power meter."

PINPOINT WEAK SPOTS. To find your strengths and weaknesses, Coggan suggests figuring average wattages for intervals of 5 seconds, 1 minute, 5 minutes, and 20 minutes. Can you hold a steady 300-watt average for 20 minutes, but will you explode if you have to pull harder than that? Maybe you can complete 20-minute efforts like an experienced racer, but your 5-minute power numbers resemble those of a beginner.

SHARPEN YOUR SPIN. If you see your watts fall dramatically when pushing a big gear or while spinning small gears, you can incorporate low-cadence/high-force or fast pedaling drills into your routine to strengthen your stroke.

GO AERO. Ride on a flat road at a steady speed, then experiment with body positions and watch your watts, says power expert Allen Lim, PhD, a sports physiology expert and coauthor of *The Feedzone Cookbook*. "You can save 25 watts and maintain your speed just by tucking," says Lim, who has calculated that a rider can shave 3:06 off a 40-kilometer time trial by shifting from the hoods to the drops, and another 2:30 by using an aerobar.

TEST IT

Power testing ranges from 30-second sprints to hour-long time trials. The most informative option: an average power profile based on all-out efforts lasting 5 seconds, 1 minute, 5 minutes, and 60 minutes. Coaches will do the test for about $75. One figure you'll want to be sure to get is your *threshold power*, a vital measurement of how much power you can sustainably produce over a 1-hour period and a fundamental metric of fitness. Threshold power is often expressed in watts produced per kilogram of body weight.

Want to test your own? Use a bike-mounted power meter, which start at around $800, or a power-enabled stationary trainer like the Wahoo KICKR. The protocol is a 20-minute all-out time trial, typically on a steady climb. Pros often do a specific series of tests that ensures better accuracy. After a 45-minute warm-up, do maximal efforts in the following order with full recovery (5–10 minutes very easy pedaling) in between each effort: 5 seconds (peak neuromuscular power), 5 minutes (peak aerobic power), 20 minutes (threshold power), and 1 minute (peak anaerobic capacity). Your functional threshold power is 95 percent of your 20-minute power number. Neal Henderson, of APEX Coaching in Boulder, Colorado, says that the threshold test must be preceded by the peak aerobic power test, or it will skew high.

SEE HOW YOU STACK UP

By comparing your power profile with those of other cyclists or to published benchmarks, you can assess your strengths and weaknesses. Above average at 1 minute but below average at 20? Work on endurance. If your power profile reveals some hidden sprinting talent, why not try a race that invites you to channel your inner Cavendish?

Here are typical power outputs for professional and fit recreational riders. Go to Bicycling.com/power for a chart that ranks power outputs for all levels of cyclists, from "untrained" to "world-class."

TIME	WATTS	
	PROFESSIONAL RIDERS (MEN/WOMEN)*	RECREATIONAL RIDERS (MEN/WOMEN)**
10 seconds	1,200+ / 900+	500+ / 400+
4–8 minutes	450 / 325	250 / 200
20–40 minutes	375 / 275	200 / 150
1–2 hours	325 / 200	175 / 120
2–4 hours	225 / 125	125 / 80

*Source: Allen Lim, PhD, sports physiology expert and coauthor of The Feedzone Cookbook.

**Source: James Herrera, owner of Performance Driven coaching, Colorado Springs, Colorado.

Get in the Zone

Once you've tested yourself, it's time to use your results to calculate your training zones. Seven zones have been specified, and different zones are emphasized throughout the year (see Training Zones chart). "The ranges allow you to know what system you're working on," Carmichael explains. "For instance, if you want to burn fat and work on fuel utilization, then you better not be working above 70 percent of your maximum heart rate because that's the point where you begin to burn carbohydrate. Most people just ride as hard as they can. But by tailoring your workout to these ranges, you'll be able to meet the objectives of your training."

TRAINING ZONES

LEVEL	NAME/PURPOSE	% OF THRESHOLD	% OF THRESHOLD HEART RATE	RATE OF PERCEIVED EXERTION	TIME
1	Active recovery	> 55%	< 68%	< 2	30 minutes– 1.5 hours
2	Endurance	56%–75%	69%–83%	2–3	1.5 hours–6 hours
3	Tempo	76%–90%	84%–94%	3–4	45 minutes– 2 hours
4	Lactate threshold	91%–105%	95%–105%	4–5	10–60 minutes
5	Maximum VO_2	106%–120%	> 106%	6–7	3–8 minutes
6	Anaerobic capacity	121%–150%	N/A	> 7	30 seconds– 3 minutes
7	Neuromuscular power	N/A	N/A	(maximal)	5–15 seconds

KEY TO THE ZONES

ZONE 1. ACTIVE RECOVERY: An embarrassingly slow pace. When you go out for a recovery ride, it should really be slow and all about recovery. If you go above the upper limit of wattage for this range, you are riding too hard.

ZONE 2. ENDURANCE: This is the level you ride at to build a base of endurance and enhance your aerobic fitness.

ZONE 3. TEMPO (OR FARTLEK): Fartlek is from Swedish, meaning "speed play." These workouts are performed at an intensity that is "up-tempo" from what a rider normally trains at when riding at a comfortable level. *Note*: The "sweet spot" is a small area of intensity characterized by 88 to 93 percent of one's functional threshold power (the maximum wattage you can sustain for one hour).

ZONE 4. LACTATE THRESHOLD: The exercise intensity at which the release of lactate into the blood first begins to exceed its rate of removal, such that blood lactate levels begin to rise.

ZONE 5. MAXIMUM VO_2: The maximal rate of whole-body oxygen uptake that can be achieved during exercise. Maximum VO_2 is primarily limited by the ability of the cardiovascular system to deliver oxygen-carrying blood to exercising muscle; hence, maximum VO_2 is considered the best measure of a person's cardiovascular fitness and sets the upper limit to aerobic power production.

ZONE 6. ANAEROBIC CAPACITY: The overall quantity of work (not the rate of doing such work, which is power) that you can perform by relying on anaerobic metabolism. Usually trained by performing short (e.g., 30-second to 3-minute), very high-intensity intervals.

ZONE 7. NEUROMUSCULAR POWER: These exercises are super-short, high-intensity efforts usually lasting less than 10 seconds each. They place a larger load on the musculoskeletal system than on the metabolic systems. You want to perform these workouts when you are the most "fresh" during the week, as the intensity of the workout is very high and you will need to be highly energized for them.

BEWARE OF DEAD ZONE SYNDROME

This condition, common among cyclists, is brought on by repeated training at a single, moderately hard intensity, known as zone 3. It afflicts enthusiasts who push the pedals hard but don't follow a training program, as well as amateur racers who have the great Eddy Merckx's famous maxim, "ride lots," indelibly burned into their brains.

SYMPTOMS AND SIGNS: Those suffering from the malady may not be aware of it, due to the syndrome's insidious nature. That's because, at a minimum, it maintains fitness, says Henderson: "You're sweating, you burn calories and you get good endurance out of it." A former hard case himself, Henderson is best known for coaching Taylor Phinney to a spot on the US Olympic team in Beijing. Many of his clients are former sufferers.

Dead zone syndrome often strikes in summer, after the body has reaped as much training benefit as possible from single-zone riding. It can manifest as a feeling of monotony, both physical and psychological. "Moderate-level intensity provides a constant stimulus to your sympathetic nervous system, your 'fight or flight' response," Henderson explains. "So if you're stressing that system to the same degree day-to-day, there'll be less recovery." In other words, you're wearing yourself down.

"You're working kind of hard, but not doing a lot to change your physiology," Henderson says. In order for your body to adapt and improve, you need to follow a program that hits the extremes, he says, especially the high end.

Pro Tip

UNPLUG ONCE IN A WHILE. Studies show that perceived exertion matches heart rate pretty spot-on. For 1 week, ride without relying on your heart rate monitor and mentally note how you feel. Later, compare your observations with actual data to get in tune with what's happening at every level of exertion.

More Lessons from the Lab

Pro cyclists let themselves be poked and prodded like lab rats for good reason: Physiological and biomechanical testing can explain how the body reacts to training and riding—and pinpoint ways to improve. Here are two more options you might want to try.

DUAL X-RAY ABSORPTIOMETRY (DXA) SCAN

WHAT: A type of X-ray that measures bone density. Cyclists tend to have lower bone density than runners, weight lifters, even sedentary people, according to University of Missouri researcher Pamela Hinton, PhD.

WHERE AND HOW MUCH: Hospitals or doctor's offices. Your health insurance may cover it; otherwise, expect to shell out about $250.

USE THE RESULTS: Build your bones by jumping. The optimal dose is 40 to 100 jarring impacts at a time. Bone doesn't respond beyond that point until it has recovered for at least 8 hours, Hinton says. Start with 20 two-legged hops three times a week and progress to single-legged hops and more repetitions.

DYNAMIC BIKE FIT

WHAT: Using computerized pedal stroke analysis, 3-D video, and laser alignment, certified fitters can tailor how your bike fits while your body is in riding motion.

WHERE AND HOW MUCH: Look for fitters certified by programs like Serotta or Retül. Pedal stroke analysis starts at $50, and a comprehensive fit runs from $200 to $300.

USE THE RESULTS: "The three pillars of proper fit are comfort, power, and aerodynamics," says Matt Russ, owner of The Sport Factory Performance Center and a certified bike fitter in Roswell, Georgia. Adjusting the fit will help you ride more efficiently and comfortably and can address unique biomechanical issues.

Pro Tip

SKIP THE MAXIMUM VO2 TEST. Scientists say the lactate threshold test is a better performance predictor.

What's Your Muscle Type?

There are two muscle types: slow twitch and fast twitch. The best way to know if you have mostly one type or the other is with a muscle biopsy—poking a hole in your leg and taking a small muscle sample. You can avoid a biopsy and get a good guess with a vertical jump test, says Harvey Newton, former adviser to the Olympic cycling team and creator of the *Strength Training for Cyclists* videos. Here's what to do:

- Warm up on a trainer for 5 to 10 minutes.

- Smear some colored chalk on your fingertips.

- Stand next to a wall, feet flat on the ground. Reach as high as you can with one hand. Mark the spot.

- Bend your legs and leap as high as possible, touching the wall and marking the spot at the highest point. Use the measurement from your best of three jumps.

The difference between the two marks is your vertical jump. Above 24 inches means you're mostly fast twitch; below it, slow twitch.

MUSCLE FIBER: FAST TWITCH

ADVANTAGE: Speed

WHAT YOU LACK: Aerobic capacity

HOW TO GET IT: Take at least one 2- to 4-hour ride per week, spending 90 to 95 percent of the ride at your 70 percent maximum heart rate.

MUSCLE FIBER: SLOW TWITCH

ADVANTAGE: Efficient oxygen output

WHAT YOU LACK: Short bursts of speed

HOW TO GET IT: Do one or two sprint workouts per week. An easy drill: Roll up to about 15 mph, stand out of the saddle, and accelerate to max speed. Sit and maintain a high speed and cadence (about 110 rpm) for 200 yards or 10 seconds. Recover 5 to 10 minutes. Repeat three to six times.

Lungs

If you could hang your lungs on a stand, you'd see spongy, elastic organs that expand and constrict as you breathe. The lungs' primary job is to draw in oxygen-rich air and expel the carbon dioxide waste generated from your cells. That exchange happens in the *alveoli*, the microscopic grape-shaped sacs that line your lungs. As you inhale normally, about half a liter of air goes in, partially filling your lungs, like a tire tube with just enough air to take shape. The air passes over the alveoli, where fresh oxygen is swapped for carbon dioxide from the bloodstream. You exhale, dump out the waste, and start again. Typically, during normal breathing, we use 10 to 15 percent of our lungs, leaving scores of alveoli untouched. Even during exercise, when we need more oxygen, we tend to get it by breathing faster—huffing and puffing—not by breathing deeper, says Paul Davenport, PhD, pulmonary researcher and professor at the University of Florida in Gainesville.

Mostly, shallow breathing is habit—it's how our body is accustomed to meeting our oxygen needs. We also unconsciously resist breathing deeply because, for most of us, it's less efficient, says Davenport. "When you breathe deep, you definitely access unused alveoli and get a greater oxygen exchange per breath. But it's more work and uses more of your body's energy." Think of inflating a tire. Filling it to 80 psi is a breeze, but as you approach 110 psi, you have to force the pump harder for each extra pound. Take a full breath. Now consciously pull more air in, filling your lungs entirely. Not easy.

ON-THE-BIKE LUNG TEST

Eric Harr, author of *Triathlon Training in Four Hours a Week*, performs this quick breathing test every few weeks to gauge his lung power. "I can now get up my test hill taking 5 breaths per minute, or about 25 breaths," says Harr.

1. Start with a 15-minute warm-up.

2. On a hill that takes about 5 minutes to climb, count how many breaths (one inhale, one exhale) it takes to reach the top.

3. Each time you take the test (optimally under similar weather conditions), try to do it in fewer breaths.

The secret to fuller, more fruitful breathing is training your lungs: forging stronger breathing habits and conditioning your respiratory muscles to make pulling in those extra liters easier. The following four tips will help you breathe better and ride stronger.

1. **BLOW IT OUT.** Encourage deeper inhalations by concentrating on full, strong exhalations that fully expel carbon dioxide from your lungs, says Harr. "Blow out your breath to a count of 3, and inhale to a count of 2. As you do it more frequently, it will become easier and more natural."

2. **BELLY BREATHE.** Concentrate on breathing deep into your body, pushing the abdominal part of your lungs down and out. Your abs should expand as much if not more than your chest, says Harr.

3. **WIDER IS BETTER.** Your body position affects how much air you can easily take in. "When you're stretched out, like on a road bike, you have a better distribution of oxygen across your lungs," says Davenport. Likewise, when your chest is open, it can more easily expand to let air in, according to Harr. "I recommend a wide bar, 2 cm wider than you'd normally ride, to help open the lungs."

4. **SYNCHRONIZE YOUR BREATHING.** "You can achieve a small increase in performance by synchronizing your breathing to your pedal stroke," says Davenport. Get into a cadence in which you're exhaling at the top of your pedal strokes, alternating legs, pushing out your air to the rhythm of your effort. You're less likely to take incomplete breaths, and your effort will feel more even.

Deep breathing can train your brain and body to make the most of your lung capacity, according to Harr. Here's one technique:

1. Sit up straight and lightly rest your hands on your stomach.

2. Breathe in through your nose for 10 seconds, expanding your lungs down and out.

3. When you've fully inhaled, breathe in a little more, then a little more. Hold that breath for 3 seconds.

4. Exhale slowly out of your mouth to a count of 5 seconds or more.

5. Repeat for 20 to 30 breaths.

Efficiency

There's another number that has nothing to do with miles per hour. Or heart rate. Or watts—though sometimes I feel as if my max might be that low. The number I'm exulting over is a new bedrock of training: *efficiency*. Vastly simplified, the term refers to the percentage of energy your body produces that actually ends up moving your bike forward. Following the same technological trickle-down as heart rate and wattage as well as other physiological markers, such as resting metabolism and body fat, efficiency was formerly measurable only under strict conditions in laboratories stocked with multimillion-dollar equipment. It is now accessible to everyday riders—in this case, using the Polar CS600 with Power cycling computer.

If you think your heart rate or wattage numbers were humbling, get ready for new levels of reality: When it comes to propulsion on a bike, we humans are horribly inefficient. According to Juuso Nissila, a physiologist formerly at Polar who helped develop the CS600 system, most amateur riders are 17 to 20 percent efficient. At either extreme, rank beginners are 17 percent or less, and many pro racers reach 22 to 23 percent.

Most of the 75 to 80 percent of our squandered energy is lost as heat. Some of it is mechanical inefficiency, like when your knee wobbles or your ankle deflects. Some of it happens when you turn your head to look at a dog, bob your shoulders, or even blink your eyes. Some of it is lost in still-undefined processes, such as various chemical reactions within your body.

Despite the small numbers, efficiency is important for three reasons.

1. It incorporates all the measurements—everything our bodies do on a bike—into one easily understood number that tells how good you are at making a bike roll. It's a simplification similar to the Apgar score for newborns or Robert Parker's wine ratings.

2. Efficiency shows you how to train away your weakness. For instance, if you produce relatively few watts but can hang with the fast group, or always finish in or near the lead group but never strongly, you are probably efficient but underpowered and need to develop more wattage. A rider who produces a lot of watts but still has trouble finishing with the lead group or otherwise underperforms—wins intermediate town sign sprints, for instance, but not the last few—is probably strong but very inefficient.

3. At the pro level, efficiency is the next frontier. With today's training, nutrition, and technology, pro racers are topping out their maximum VO$_2$ and watt-producing abilities. For them, raising efficiency a single percentage point could be worth hundreds of thousands of dollars in performance gains. For pro and recreational riders alike, a 2 percent gain in efficiency is huge and may take a season or more to achieve because the nature of efficiency is broad and ambiguous. You might gain efficiency by pedaling a different way (a change in cadence, saddle height, foot position, or how you activate your muscles), by changing your body position, or by relaxing more—it takes a lot of trial and error.

Because efficiency includes not only your body's performance but how the bike and body interact, the monitor can tell you which components are more efficient for you (for instance, if you swap wheels and your efficiency rises). This works from handlebar to saddle to pedals.

Don't be fooled: Being efficient doesn't mean you're faster, only that you're moving the bike more economically. The payoff is that you save power for when you need to dig deep. Polar scientists say they've seen one racer at 25 percent efficiency and have reviewed a study of a climber who reached 27 percent. "It doesn't seem possible to go beyond that," says Nissila. That doesn't mean I can't keep trying. Unlike wattage at threshold or a 40K time trial time, efficiency is the measurement that you have the best chance of raising to a pro level—or better.

THE SIMPLEST WAY TO GAIN EFFICIENCY

All that breakthrough tech talk is exciting stuff—but when it comes to efficiency, most of us benefit from a simpler worldview: We just need to find more time to ride. Here are four tips that really work.

1. **GET UP 70 MINUTES EARLIER.** That's 10 minutes to dodder about and 1 hour to ride. You will suffer for 3 weeks, but then it will become ingrained.

2. **CLIMB.** The 13-mile Churchview hill ride near *Bicycling* headquarters is a tougher

workout than the 21-mile Sauerkraut Long flat ride.

3. **PREP IN ADVANCE.** After each ride, wipe and lube the chain and inflate the tires 5 psi over the recommendation—next morning you can hop on and go.

4. **COMMIT.** Schedule rides with a friend—even when, inevitably, time becomes crunched, you'll be less likely to blow off a ride if you know someone's waiting for you.

PART II

PREP

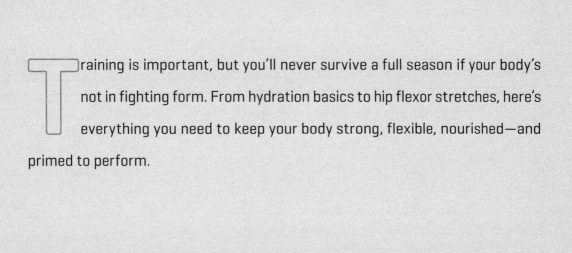

Training is important, but you'll never survive a full season if your body's not in fighting form. From hydration basics to hip flexor stretches, here's everything you need to keep your body strong, flexible, nourished—and primed to perform.

CHAPTER 4

Nutrition and Hydration

It's okay to eat almost anything you want as long as you do not eat too much of it. Remember that you will pay for everything. If you eat too many grams of fat you must train that much more to get rid of them.

—TONY ROMINGER, RETIRED SWISS PROFESSIONAL ROAD RACER

FROM LIGHTER BIKES TO AERO HELMETS TO INTERVAL-HEAVY training programs, cyclists look for every edge to get faster. The irony is, they often overlook the one thing that delivers performance benefits without so much as a single crank of the pedals: food. Sure, food fuels you through your workouts, but beyond delivering calories it offers a spectrum of ride-boosting benefits spanning everything from livelier muscles to faster recovery between workouts—even improved speed. "Food truly can be a performance enhancer," says Iñigo San Millán, PhD, a world-renowned exercise physiologist and the director of the Human Performance Laboratory at the University of Colorado's Anschutz Health and Wellness Center in Denver. "Only part of food's benefit is the energy you get. The rest is its nutrients, because those can also improve your performance." You just have to know how to squeeze the greatest benefits from every plate of food—and that means knowing not only what to eat, but also when to eat it. In this chapter, we'll take a look at the building blocks of your diet—carbohydrates, protein, fat, fluids, and their many forms—and discuss how to carry this nutritional knowledge onto the bike.

Carbs

For the last 40 years, carbohydrates have been accused of a laundry list of crimes against humanity, including multiple counts of conspiracy to make us fat. This is partly because too many of us fill our bellies with the wrong kinds—breads, chips, crackers, and pastas made from refined flour that's been processed to within an inch of its nutritional life. Cyclists in particular have also gotten confusing messages about carbs thanks to trends like the protein-centric, grain-shunning Paleo diet and from pro riders who have gone public about going gluten free. All this has many of us pedaling scared from an essential fuel source that makes us faster, fitter, and smarter on the bike. Harnessing the power of the carbohydrate is not as simple as stocking a pantry full of bagels and filling your bottles with sports drinks. To understand why, you first need to consider these three irrefutable facts.

FACT: Carbs make you a speedier, savvier rider—and may even help you get leaner.

Your body uses carbs to make glucose, or blood sugar, the fuel that drives athletic performance. Within limits, "the more carbohy-

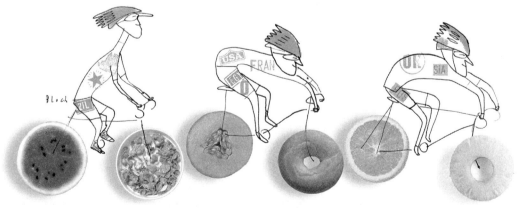

Carbs are the nutrients that power your rides.

drates you consume during endurance exercise, the better you perform," says sports nutrition researcher Asker Jeukendrup, PhD, global senior director of the Gatorade Sports Science Institute. In a study of endurance cyclists completing a 238-mile race, those who took in the most carbs (the mean was 52 grams per hour for the 16-hour event) posted the fastest times. And the benefits go well beyond performance. "All systems and tissues in your body use carbohydrates in some capacity," says Stacy T. Sims, PhD, an exercise physiologist and nutrition scientist at the Stanford Prevention Research Center who has consulted for pro cycling teams. Carbs fuel your immune system and brain, enhance fluid absorption so you stay hydrated, and are even critical for muscle recovery. In fact, if you fail to feed your body the carbs it needs, it will generate them by breaking down muscle tissue.

FACT: Not all carbs are created equal, but there's a time and place for most of them.

Carbohydrates fall into two categories, simple and complex. Simple carbs are made from one or two sugars, like fructose or glucose. They're found in such sweeteners as cane sugar, corn syrup, maple syrup, brown sugar, and honey. Because your body digests them quickly, they trigger a quick surge in insulin, the hormone that ushers glucose from your bloodstream into your cells to fuel activity. Refined and processed foods like white bread,

white pasta, cakes, and pastries also fall into this category because they're stripped of fiber and other compounds that slow digestion and the insulin response. Simple carbs get a bad rap because sudden spikes and falls in blood sugar have been linked to overeating and, subsequently, to increased fat storage.

Complex carbohydrates are made from more than two sugar molecules and take longer to break down in your body, so you have a more measured blood sugar and insulin response. Complex carbs tend to contain fiber, which also slows digestion. About 50 percent of your total calorie intake should come from carbs, primarily the complex variety, says Michigan-based sports dietitian Donna Marlor, RD, CSSD. Carbs like fruits, vegetables, legumes, and whole grains are lower in calories, digest more slowly, and contain vitamins, minerals, and immunity-boosting phytonutrients.

Simple carbs also have a place, especially before and during rides when you need quick energy. The good news is that because you're a cyclist, your body is primed to digest and use these carbs while exercising. Muscle contraction stimulates a special protein that transports glucose directly into your cells without insulin's help, says Marlor.

FACT: When you're riding, your digestive system can handle more than you think.

Scientists used to say the body can absorb a maximum of 30 to 60 grams of carbs an hour, or one gram a minute, during exercise. Jeuken-drup's lab has found that athletes can digest more if they take in more than one kind of carb. Remember the different types of simple sugars? Turns out you have individual trans-porters in your gut that break down each type and shuttle it to your bloodstream. These transporters can absorb only a fixed amount in a given time period. So if your glucose transporters are maxed out at 60 grams, oth-ers, like those for fructose, are still available. In tests, "we were able to increase carbohy-drate absorption up to 1.75 grams a minute with a drink blend that included fructose,"

SHOULD YOU GO GLUTEN FREE?

IN 2008 ALLEN LIM, PHD, SPORTS PHYSIOLOGY expert and coauthor of *The Feedzone Cookbook*, announced that his Garmin–Slipstream riders were going wheat free (goodbye pasta and bread) because gluten—a protein in wheat grain—might interfere with digestion. Since then, performance-minded cyclists of all levels started ditching the stuff. While Lim's squad swapped their wheat-based noodles and starches for healthy gluten-free grains like rice, oats, and quinoa, many everyday riders simply stocked up on commercially altered gluten-free foods, such as scones, cookies, and breads. "These are highly processed foods filled with gums, additives, and processed grains, which aren't any better for you," says Stacy T. Sims, PhD, an exercise physiologist and nutrition scientist at the Stanford Prevention Research Center.

There certainly are legitimate reasons to give up gluten. Some people have celiac disease, an inability to digest the protein, which leads to gastrointestinal distress; others may have wheat allergies. A doctor can test you for both conditions. Some experts say you can simply have a gluten sensitivity, which may hamper digestion without causing more overt symptoms. The only way to test for gluten sensitivity is to stop eating gluten and see how you feel. "Be sure to substitute in unprocessed grains like amaranth and quinoa, not just 'gluten-free' processed foods," says Sims.

The bottom line is that athletes who have no discernible symptoms likely won't see performance gains from giving up gluten and will miss out on the slow-burning carbs and nutrients in wheat, especially the whole grain variety. As Marlor says, "It's an important part of an athlete's diet."

WHAT CYCLISTS NEED TO KNOW ABOUT THE PALEO DIET

LET'S SAY YOU WANT TO TAKE YOUR everyday diet back to the Stone Age and subsist on lean meats, fruits, and vegetables (no grains, legumes, or dairy) for most meals, as advocated by the popular Paleo diet. The fact is, you cannot perform at a high level without the fast-acting carbohydrates that high-carb foods provide. Even the diet's creators recognize this. In their book *The Paleo Diet for Athletes*, authors Loren Cordain and Joe Friel concede that endurance athletes need to "bend the rules" and eat "nonoptimal foods," such as bread, pasta, bagels, rice, corn, and other items rich in glucose, to fuel their efforts and promote full recovery, before, during, and after exercise. As with most of these diets, you'll still wind up eating less processed crap. "If you eat 'clean' and low on the food chain," says Sims, "your body is going to respond well."

says Jeukendrup. That's more than 400 calories an hour.

You need to train your system to handle that amount of fuel, however. "If you only eat 200 or 250 calories an hour in training, your gut won't suddenly accept twice that much during a race," says Jeukendrup. You need to gradually increase your carb intake during training to get in the range of 400. The trick is to meter it out instead of dumping it all in at once. If you're riding longer than an hour and a half, eat every 20 minutes and drink every 15 minutes. Just 30 to 60 grams an hour is fine for easy jaunts. For longer, harder efforts, aim for about 80 grams, says Marlor.

Sims recommends getting most of those carbs from food, with just 20 grams (about 80 calories' worth) in your bottles to improve hydration without bogging down your belly. And look for drinks that contain a mixture of two or more carbohydrates, like glucose, fructose, or sucrose.

66

Percent increase in stored glycogen when you eat carbs along with caffeine, according to the *Journal of Applied Physiology.*

SUGAR SHOCK

The fact that your body needs simple sugars while riding doesn't give you have free rein to eat them off the bike. They're bad for your arteries and organs when you do a lot of sitting around. And even though cyclists are more active than people who don't exercise, many of us spend more time at our desks (or on couches) than we do in our saddles. During inactivity, the sugar your muscles would normally sponge up forces your body to secrete insulin, the metabolic doorman that escorts free-floating sugar from your bloodstream into your cells. The doorman can work only so fast, however. If you pour in too much sugar, insulin starts blocking it, leaving it in your bloodstream, where it latches onto proteins and damages blood vessel walls. That leads to inflammation, which paves the way for hardened arteries and heart disease. In the meantime, your body still pumps out insulin to try to clean up the mess and eventually converts the excess glucose into stored fat. Repeat this process over and over again, and the doorman eventually calls it quits, which means you can no longer get sugar into your cells, and that signals diabetes.

Eating a sugar bomb (a slice of cake, a doughnut) also triggers blood sugar fluctuations and imbalances of the hormones that regulate appetite, which can lead to overeating and fat gain, especially in your belly. Some experts, most notably Joe Friel, author of *The Cyclist's Training Bible* and *The Paleo Diet for Athletes*, caution that eating a lot of sugar in your daily diet also hinders your fat-burning metabolism both on and off the bike, so you're less efficient in training. "Your body is very adaptive," says Friel. "It'll use what you give it the most of. And the more sugar that comes in, the more your body attunes to using quick energy." That means you don't burn fat as readily for fuel, which leads to faster energy drain.

Not only does consuming excess sugar alter your fat-burning metabolism, it also changes your brain circuitry and may even be addictive. That's right: There's a reason you "can't eat just one." Sugar lights up the same reward receptors and triggers the same cascade of feel-good brain chemicals (like serotonin and dopamine) as cocaine does. So when you're trolling for a post-ride cookie even though you sucked down a gel during your ride, it may not be about restocking your energy stores as much as it is about feeding your head. And because overloading on sugar messes with the chemistry in areas of the brain that control food intake, it becomes harder to regulate how much we eat. So we end up eating even more sugar and get caught in a vicious cycle.

Cut out foods with added sugar from your daily menu. The most obvious are sodas, bakery goods, and candy. But as noted earlier, you'll also find sugar in most processed foods that come in a box, jar, carton, or can. Watch for added sugar in a multitude of names and incarnations, including beet sugar, corn sugar, corn sweetener, corn syrup, fruit juice concentrate or puree, high-fructose corn syrup, honey, malt sugar, molasses, syrup, and maple syrup. Ingredients ending in *ose* are all forms of sugar. If any of those are among the first three to five on the list of ingredients, that's too much sugar.

YOUR DAILY CARBS

Just as you wouldn't buy a bunch of perishable food before leaving on a vacation, you don't need to consume hundreds of grams of carbs if you're doing nothing more strenuous than tapping a keyboard. Sims recommends these guidelines for matching your overall daily carb intake to how much activity you do. Each gram of carbohydrate provides four calories of energy.

EXERCISE LEVEL	RECOMMENDED DAILY CARBOHYDRATES*
Low/easy	205–275 grams (less than 1 hour a day)
Moderate	275–340 grams (about 1 hour a day)
Very active	410–475 grams (1–3 hours a day)
Extremely active	545–580 grams (4–5 hours a day or more)

*Recommendations are for a 150-pound cyclist.

Protein

Skimp on protein, and your body borrows from muscle to meet its needs—undermining the fitness you've worked so hard to achieve. "Getting enough protein protects your lean mass," says Roberta Anding, RD, clinical dietitian and director of sports nutrition in the department of pediatrics, adolescent medicine, and sports medicine at Texas Children's Hospital in Houston. "And that's where the power in your ride comes from."

Because protein slows digestion and lowers a food's rating on the glycemic index, it prevents high-energy carbs from sending your blood sugar soaring, then crashing. That's especially valuable during long days in the saddle, when steady-release energy keeps you from bonking. During fuel shortages, your body sends protein to the liver, where it gets turned into backup carbs.

The power of protein doesn't stop there. Its amino acids act like recovery agents that refresh your body for the next go-round: After a muscle-ravaging ride, protein rebuilds tissues and prepares them for more. It also bolsters the immune system; our bodies require protein to make infection-fighting white blood cells.

Anding recommends that cyclists consume

FOR WOMEN ONLY

REMEMBER TO GET ENOUGH IRON, ESPECIALLY IF your training program represents a significant increase in training load. A premenopausal woman's daily requirement for iron is 18 mg, more than double that of a man, and this requirement balloons to 33 mg for premenopausal vegetarian women. Iron is a crucial component of oxygen-carrying hemoglobin. Fortunately it's easy to meet these requirements without resorting to supplements. Foods rich in iron include:

TOFU: 13 mg in ½ cup of firm style tofu

FORTIFIED BREAKFAST CEREALS: 5 to 16 mg in a ¾ cup serving, depending on the brand

BEANS: 5 to 7 mg per cup, depending on the bean

LEAN BEEF: roughly 1 mg per ounce

a daily dose of 0.5 to 0.6 grams of protein per pound of body weight—that's about 85 grams for a 170-pound rider. Eat 15 to 25 grams of that during recovery within an hour of finishing a ride. And always target lean sources. "Skip the animal proteins that are loaded with saturated fats, such as full-fat cheeses and burgers, and opt for reduced-fat dairy or lean meats," Anding says. Here's how to maximize your protein intake—without unwanted calories.

KNOW THE SCORE

High-quality protein sources offer more muscle-building amino acids than others, and thus are more valuable to cyclists. "Eggs and dairy products are incredibly high-quality sources," says Anding. Such proteins are considered "complete" because they contain enough of all the essential amino acids needed to rebuild cells. Milk is particularly high in branched-chain amino acids, including leucine, which has been found to trigger muscle recovery.

Except for certain grains, such as quinoa, most plant proteins are "incomplete," or lack a few key amino acids. "To build and repair tissue, those proteins need a little help," Anding says. Traditional food pairings often form complete combos: Beans are good, but adding rice increases the overall protein quality.

Proteins are absorbed at different rates

(similar to fast- and slow-release carbs). Whey, a milk protein, is digested quickly, which is why it's preferred in recovery beverages. Another milk protein, casein, is slowly digested, so it's ideal for minimizing blood sugar spikes throughout the day.

DOUBLE UP

Choose protein sources that are also high in other valuable nutrients. Lean beef and dark meat chicken (legs and thighs) contain high-quality protein and iron, which help deliver oxygen to working muscles. Coldwater fish (such as cod and salmon) pair protein with omega-3 fatty acids—anti-inflammatory agents that ease aching joints and over-worked muscles. Many low-fat dairy products combine big doses of protein (28 grams in one cup of cottage cheese) with calcium, which stimulates muscle contraction and keeps muscles firing.

Fat

Protein may be the diet du jour, but if you're in search of a real cycling boost, get fat. New evidence shows that the right kind of dietary fat not only fuels you on long rides but also may help you lose weight, build muscle, and recover faster. What's more, it's good for your heart, the engine that keeps those pistons pumping.

There are different types of fat. Good fats include: monounsaturated, such as those from fish oil, olive oil, egg yolks, and peanut butter; and polyunsaturated (especially omega-3 fatty acids), such as those from nuts and fish. Bad or neutral fats include: saturated, such as those from animal and coconut fats; and the worst kind, trans fats, the man-made fats found in margarine, cookies, chips, and fries. The goal is to get more of the good—about one-third of your diet—and less of the bad.

"Studies show that higher fat diets make more sense for fit people than low-fat diets," says nutritionist Liz Applegate, PhD, author of *Encyclopedia of Sports and Fitness Nutrition*. "In one study, endurance athletes ran up to 24 percent longer before they fatigued when they ate a diet that was above 30 percent fat compared to one that was below 20 percent," she says.

One of the surprising benefits of eating dietary fat that researchers are just now beginning to grasp is that it burns body fat. Recent research shows that omega-3 fatty acids, a type of polyunsaturated fat found in flaxseed and fish oil, increases the size of your cells' fuel-burning furnaces and raises your metabolic rate, causing you to burn more calories every minute of every day. Omega-3s also help make you more sensitive to insulin, the chemical your body releases after you eat to help push food into storage. Being sensitive to insulin ultimately means you store less fat and the fat that you do have stocked away is more easily used as energy. The result is healthy blood sugar and an appetite free of sugar spikes, crashes, and cravings. Omega-3 fats also help generate testosterone, the hormone we need for muscle building. More muscle plus more calorie burning equals less body fat.

Fat also helps your heart. Monounsaturated fats are known to help lower bad LDL cholesterol, and omega-3 fatty acids make your blood as slippery as the fish they come from to prevent blood clots, so your heart can do its job without stress or strain.

Finally, fat may help you recover faster from your leg-ripping rides. Important muscle-repairing, bone-building antioxidant vitamins such as A, D, E, and K are fat soluble. That means eating fat helps usher more of these essential nutrients from your intestines into your bloodstream where they can work their magic. "There's evidence that 1 to 1.5 grams of omega-3 fatty acids a day help reduce muscle pain in active people," says Applegate. "I recommend eating a fatty fish, such as salmon, twice a week to get all the benefits of these healthy fats."

Experts recommend getting 7 to 11 grams of omega-3 fatty acids each week—something few meat-and-potato-loving Americans accomplish. Here are the top omega-3–containing foods. Eat just one or two a day, and you'll meet your mark.

FOOD	PORTION	TOTAL OMEGA-3S (GRAMS)*
Flaxseed oil	1 Tbsp	6.9
Walnuts	1 oz	2.6
Salmon, canned (drained)	4 oz	2.2
Sardines, canned (drained)	4 oz	1.8
Salmon, fresh or frozen	4 oz	1.7
Canola oil	1 Tbsp	1.3
Cod, fresh or frozen	4 oz	0.6
Crab, soft shell, cooked	4 oz	0.6
Scallops, Maine, fresh or frozen, cooked	4 oz	0.5
Soybeans, dried, cooked	½ c	0.5

Source: Minnesota Nutrient Data Base 4:04

Build a Better Diet

To make the best use of carbs, fats, and protein, trade your typical Western diet for something a bit more exotic. In the region where olives flourish, people flourish, too. Heart disease, cancer, diabetes, and even Alzheimer disease are far less common in Mediterranean countries, such as Greece, Italy, France, and Spain. Perhaps this explains why many of the world's best bike racers have a nutritional leg up. "Mediterranean eaters place an emphasis on fresh, quality ingredients" based on the region's eating patterns, according to Cynthia Sass, MPH, RD, coauthor of *S.A.S.S. Yourself Slim*. Mediterranean dishes often build on a few flavor-packed ingredients, such as

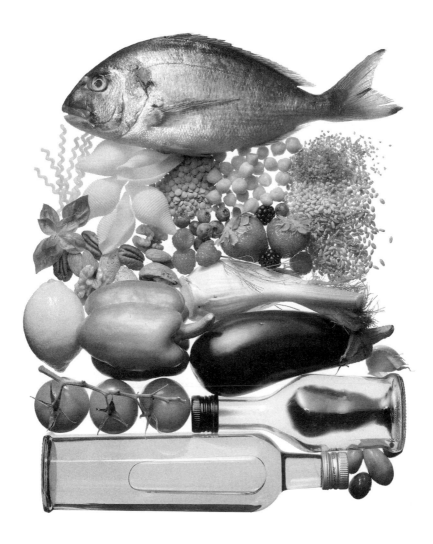

A Mediterranean diet contains an optimal mix of lean protein, healthy carbs, and good fats.

tomatoes, basil, and balsamic vinegar. Follow Sass's advice to import the best of the Mediterranean into your kitchen.

MAKE VEGGIES THE CENTERPIECE

Mediterranean meals typically consist of about 75 percent plant matter from fruits, vegetables, whole grains, and beans. "Meat is considered a condiment and is eaten infrequently," says Sass. Greeks, for example, eat little red meat but consume an average of nine daily servings of fruits and vegetables. These proportions offer a broad spectrum of vitamins, minerals, and antioxidants, which stave off disease and fuel athletic performance.

TRY IT: Pick a vegetable or fruit and design the meal around it. Pair great berries with oatmeal or mix broccoli into a pasta sauce. Fresh, in-season fruits and veggies deliver the highest nutrient content, and you can save them for other times of the year as well. "Freezing tends to lock in nutrients and preserve them, so many frozen foods are just as nutritious as when they are fresh," says Sass.

CHOOSE PLANT-BASED FATS

Foods popular in the Mediterranean—like nuts and olive oil—aren't low in fat. But they contain monounsaturated fat, the good kind that lowers total cholesterol levels. Plus, several studies have found that the diet fosters weight loss. One 2008 paper published in the

New England Journal of Medicine reported that those who switched to a Mediterranean diet lost an average of 9.7 pounds, compared with 6.4 pounds for those who followed a low-fat diet plan.

TRY IT: Use olive oil in place of butter or mayo and snack on nuts instead of cheese. Slice an avocado into your salad or sandwich.

SEASON FOOD LIBERALLY

"Cyclists need more antioxidants in their diets to repair the wear and tear from long rides," says Sass. Mediterranean food is amply seasoned with herbs and spices so packed with antioxidants that even small doses deliver powerful benefits. One teaspoon of cinnamon delivers as many antioxidants as a cup of pomegranate juice.

TRY IT: Add antioxidant-rich herbs and spices, such as oregano, cinnamon, or dill, to entrees. Place lemon slices over fish and beans to make a zingy dish. Grow a windowsill herb garden for a supply of flavor-packed seasonings.

SWAP YOUR PROTEIN

Fish, rather than beef, is the go-to protein, so Mediterranean eaters are consuming more healthy fatty acids than artery-clogging saturated fats.

TRY IT: Sass recommends two or three seafood-based meals per week rounded out with vegetables, such as a salad of beans or greens.

FIND YOUR VEG EDGE

VEGETARIANS TAKE NOTE: A STUDY IN THE *Journal of the International Society of Sports Nutrition* concludes that cyclists who went meatless had to work harder (based on VO$_2$ measurements) to achieve the same results during a cycling test than their carnivorous peers who ate more protein. Round out a meat-free diet with plant-based protein sources. Aim for one to two servings of beans every day (about a cup per serving) as well as daily servings of soy, nuts, and whole grains, says Leslie Bonci, MPH, RD, director of sports nutrition at the University of Pittsburgh Medical Center.

EAT AWAY INFLAMMATION

Ride hard, and inflammation inevitably results: It's how the body tries to repair worked muscles and joints. Paradoxically, though, inflammation also causes soreness and slows recovery. You can always take ibuprofen, but recent research shows that some foods contain anti-inflammatory agents that ease aches and hasten healing. Eat them to fuel your workouts—and bounce back faster.

Some healthy fats, such as the omega-3 fatty acids in salmon and tuna, are one example. University of Pittsburgh Medical Center researchers found that omega-3s relieved joint pain in 60 percent of subjects, and a study published in the March 2009 *Clinical Journal of Sport Medicine* showed that they alleviated delayed-onset muscle soreness after strenuous exercise.

Cherries and berries also contain anti-inflammatory properties, which is why Team Garmin-Transitions members down pomegranate juice after hard rides. One study published in the *British Journal of Sports Medicine* found that, after strenuous exercise, subjects who drank tart cherry juice felt less soreness and just a 4 percent strength loss the next day (compared with a 22 percent strength loss with the placebo). The spice turmeric contains curcumin, which one study found to reduce muscle inflammation and increase endurance in exercising mice.

Note that you'll benefit more from whole foods than supplements: Evidence suggests that flooding the body with antioxidants dampens its ability to make its own.

BONE UP ON CALCIUM

Cyclists know that carbs fuel performance—but does calcium? Like sodium and potassium, this mineral plays a supporting role in muscle contraction, and it's lost through sweat. "If calcium isn't one of the electrolytes you're replacing, your performance could be compromised because mineral loss affects the transmission of nerve impulses and thus decreases the muscles' ability to perform," says Adam Kelinson, a nutrition consultant and author of *The Athlete's Plate*. In other words: Lose too much calcium and you lose your edge.

What's more, preliminary studies suggest that increasing calcium intake may preserve cyclists' bone mass. Long-distance riding takes a toll on bone health because the sustained stress elevates levels of the parathyroid hormone, which leaches calcium from bones. In fact, Tour de France cyclists can lose as much as 25 percent of their bone mineral density over the 3-week race. Pilot studies performed at the University of Colorado, Denver, showed that drinking calcium-enriched water before and during exercise lowered parathyroid levels by 25 percent. So calcium keeps your muscles firing strong and may shore up your skeleton, too.

Dairy products are the richest sources of absorbable calcium, but dairy fats can aggravate inflammation in various parts of the body, including joints and muscles. So go for fat-free or low-fat versions of milk and yogurt, which are both high in calcium. During rides, sip a calcium-enriched electrolyte drink.

DOSE ON D

"Years of evidence suggest that vitamin D improves athletic performance," says Bruce Hollis, PhD, professor of pediatrics, biochemistry, and molecular biology at the Medical University of South Carolina in Charleston, who coauthored a review of about 50 studies linking vitamin D to athletic enhancement in the May 2009 issue of *Medicine and Science in Sports and Exercise*. In the research he examined, athletes absorbed vitamin D through ultraviolet light or supplements—then exercised faster and stronger, and with greater endurance, than those who didn't receive vitamin D. "The Russians and Germans knew this decades ago, and used it to enhance the performance of their athletes," Hollis says. Researchers don't yet understand the exact mechanism responsible for the boost. Hollis has hypothesized that muscles' vitamin D receptors absorb the nutrient, which stimulates muscle function.

Sunlight is a great source of vitamin D. Just 20 minutes of full exposure provides up to 20,000 IU (our bodies need at least 600 IU daily, according to the National Institutes of Health). Trouble is, soaking up too much sun can lead to skin cancer, and sunscreen blocks vitamin D–producing wavelengths. Thus, experts recommend downing fortified milk, cereals, and salmon (one 4-ounce serving of sockeye salmon contains 739 IU) instead of relying on sun exposure for your daily dose of

SHOULD YOU SKIP BREAKFAST?

A SMALL STUDY ON CYCLISTS IN THE journal *Medicine and Science in Sports and Exercise* concluded that riding in a fasted state burns fat better than when you're fueled up. Breakfast skippers everywhere felt vindicated—but don't pass on the oatmeal just yet. Other studies show that endurance athletes burn equal amounts of fat regardless of whether they fasted or fueled beforehand. Plus, when you eat a little something before a ride, you get a bonus calorie burn when your body fires up its digestive juices, according to Bonci. "You can ride harder on fuel than on fumes," she says, "so you get a better workout and burn more calories overall, which is really what matters."

vitamin D. Or take a daily supplement of 1,000 to 2,000 IU, which may seem high compared with the Recommended Dietary Allowance (RDA) of 400 IU, but Hollis says that figure is outdated. "If I was a coach, I'd have all my athletes—especially dark-skinned ones—taking a supplement," he insists.

Nutritionists agree. Tara Gidus, RD, an endurance athlete and sports dietitian in Orlando, Florida, takes 2,000 IU per day. That's because vitamin D deficiency has been linked to heart disease, osteoporosis, and breast, colon, and prostate cancer—and because of the possible performance benefit.

Bar None

Before you gobble another sticky slab of food, consider this: You might not have worked out

hard enough to burn it off. "The problem is, people don't count the calories they're taking in and will eat an energy bar or a recovery bar or both, then eat a meal on top of it," says

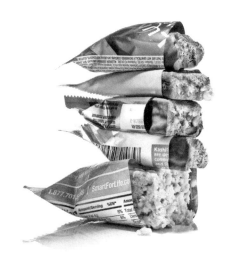

Prepackaged bars can be a convenient source of nutrients—if you choose wisely.

Cynthia Sass, MPH, RD, "Bars have their place," she says. "But you have to consider what kind of rider you are and what you want the bar to accomplish." This section outlines different bar types and how they can help, or hurt, you.

BAR: ENERGY (AKA Carbohydrate)

THE BASICS: The most crowded category in sports foods—it grew nearly 24 percent in 2004 alone. Easily digestible and specially formulated to deliver a big hit of carbs (about 40 grams, or 70 percent, of the bar's calories).

PURPOSE: Provides a steady stream of carbohydrates during your workout so you don't bonk. After your workout, such bars can replenish the glycogen that you've spent.

LOOK FOR: A high carbohydrate count and fewer than 2 grams of fiber. Your best choice is one that contains B vitamins, which are needed in combination with carbs for optimal performance.

WATCH OUT FOR: Too many calories—energy bars can pack 350 or more. Unrecognizable ingredients, especially sugar alcohols like xylitol or maltitol, which are hard to digest and can cause stomach discomfort.

BAR: RECOVERY (AKA Protein)

THE BASICS: High in muscle-building protein, these bars are marketed as much to the gym bench-pressing crowd as to the pedal-pushing cyclists looking for post-ride and post-training recovery.

PURPOSE: Helps usher carbs back into your muscles after a hard ride, and provides amino acids to rebuild your muscles. These supplements work quickly so your body begins recovery immediately.

LOOK FOR: Quality protein in the form of whey, milk, and soy. There is much debate over which is best, but many bars contain a blend, which may help deliver the benefits of each.

WATCH OUT FOR: Again, too many calories—some bars contain as many as 500 calories. These bars are essentially a small meal—one bar can have as much protein as 3 ounces of chicken and as many carbs as a cup of brown rice.

BAR: WOMEN'S

THE BASICS: Usually contain ingredients purportedly good for a woman's general health—calcium, folic acid, iron, or soy protein. They are generally lower in calories and often the go-to choice for skinny male cyclists.

PURPOSE: Provide women (as well as smaller riders) with the vitamins and minerals they need, in a low-calorie, reasonable portion.

LOOK FOR: Bars with fewer than 200 calories or minibars—half-size versions of popular bars—which usually go down in two or three bites and serve up about 100 calories.

WATCH OUT FOR: Packaging waste. Unless you need the extra calcium, iron, or other women-specific nutrients, you can simply cut your regular energy bars in half.

BAR: MEAL REPLACEMENT

THE BASICS: These "miscellaneous" bars, whether it's because of their carb count, protein content, or marketing, don't fall into the other categories.

PURPOSE: An easy way to get carbs, protein, fat, and calories in one convenient package. Some people use them as a prepackaged meal and a way to prevent mindless overeating.

LOOK FOR: Natural ingredients. Bars made from grains and fruits do a better job of simulating the nuances of a real meal, including antioxidants, vitamins, and minerals.

WATCH OUT FOR: Relying too heavily on them. Bars are a great way to fit in a meal on the go, but real food offers more variety, a wider range of nutrients and antioxidants, and will tend to be more satiating.

Hydration Basics

Cyclists, like all athletes, need plenty of liquids. Beyond that basic tenet, things get murky fast—and for years, riders have heard conflicting reports about what, when, and how much to drink. So we tapped our best resources, from the latest research to sports nutrition expert Monique Ryan, RD, author of *Sports Nutrition for Endurance Athletes*, to separate the facts from the hype. Here's what we found.

HYPE: Replace Every Lost Ounce

For years cyclists have been told to drink enough on the bike so that they weigh the same after the ride as they did beforehand. The truth is, your body can't absorb fluids as fast as it loses them, and not every ounce of weight is lost through sweat anyway.

TRUTH: Keep Up with Sweat Loss, Mostly

Replace about 75 percent of lost sweat during a long ride. "To do that, you need to know your sweat rate," says Ryan, who recently coached a heavy-sweating triathlete who routinely lost 40 ounces of fluid an hour. To determine your sweat rate, weigh yourself before and after a short ride. "An hour ride is a good indicator of what you're losing through sweat alone," Ryan says.

HYPE: Overflow Beforehand

Guzzling gallons of fluids before a ride or race will do little more than send you searching for rest stops.

TRUTH: Top Off As You Go

Sip a 16-ounce sports drink an hour or two before you saddle up. That's enough time for your body to absorb what it needs and eliminate what it doesn't. Then take in about 6 to 8 ounces (two to three gulps) every 15 to 20 minutes while you ride.

HYPE: You Need More Protein

Initially, carbohydrates were the essential building blocks of the sports beverage. Then protein muscled its way onto the scene, after early studies showed that carb–protein blends seemed to shoot into the bloodstream and

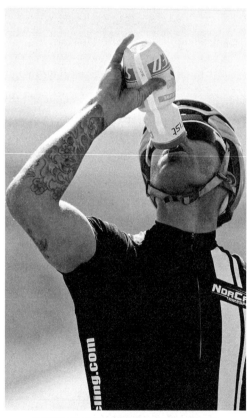

Aim to replace about 75 percent of lost sweat.

enhance endurance cycling performance better than carb-only beverages.

TRUTH: You Need a Little Protein . . . Maybe

Recent research on 10 trained cyclists performing an 80-K trial showed that riders drinking carb-only beverages did just as well as those drinking carb–protein beverages, and both groups did better than those consuming flavored water. However, the International Society of Sports Nutrition recently reported that taking in branched-chain amino acids during vigorous aerobic exercise can decrease muscle damage and depletion. "If you're on a long ride where you're also eating, you'll be taking in protein already," says Ryan, "so it's likely not necessary to also have it in your drink."

HYPE: Hydration During Exercise Is the Be-All and End-All

Big beverage companies would have you grabbing your sports drink during every ride, no matter how long or short the effort, lest you suffer the ill effects of dehydration.

TRUTH: Drinking Every Day Is Essential

"Your first priority should be staying on top of your daily hydration," says Ryan. Research on gym-goers found that nearly half began their workouts in a dehydrated state. "Many people don't consume enough fluids during the day," Ryan says. "If you hydrate properly on a regular basis, you won't need to worry as much about getting dehydrated during a typical moderate ride." The old eight-glasses-a-day dictum is a good guidepost.

10

Percentage that your performance improves when you sip cold fluids during hard rides in hot weather. Cyclists who guzzled chilled drinks finished a time trial in 90-degree heat 2 minutes faster than those whose drinks were air temperature, according to a study in the *International Journal of Sport Nutrition and Exercise Metabolism.*

STAYING HYDRATED IN THE HEAT

Sipping fluids before and after a hot-weather workout is just as important as drinking during a ride. Here we turn to the experts for the when, how, and what of staying quenched.

TIME IT RIGHT: Hydrating before pedaling helps you avoid drying out on the road. For best absorption, sip 12 to 16 ounces of water 4 hours before hopping onto your bike and sip another 12 ounces 2 hours before your ride begins. While riding, drink enough to match the intensity of the exercise, the heat of the day, and your body's needs—the average rec-

ommendation is one 16-ounce bottle per hour in cool weather and as many as four bottles per hour in extremely hot weather, based on a 150-pound cyclist. Afterward, your goal is to replace lost fluids and electrolytes. If the ride was easy or moderate, sipping water and having a small meal within an hour of finishing should be sufficient, but if the ride was long and intense, use the weighing method below to determine your drinking regimen.

CUSTOMIZE: People sweat at different rates and rides vary in terrain, speed, and distance, but hydration goals are the same regardless. "Your aim is to minimize fluid and electrolyte loss or gain," says Douglas Casa, PhD, the director of athletic training education at the University of Connecticut. Again, the best way to learn your individual sweat rate is to step on the scale before and after a long or hard ride. If you weigh less afterward, you should be drinking a bit more; if you weigh more, you should cut back to avoid overhydration.

KEEP IT SIMPLE: "On easier rides, stick with

Pro Tip

After you grab your water bottle, don't tilt your head to drink. Tilt the bottle and squeeze the water in. You'll have more control.

water. You'll get the mother lode of electrolytes, calories, and fluids from the meals and fluids you consume prior to, and after, your ride," says Casa, who's been researching hydration and exercise issues for more than a decade. When a ride is intense, pushes past an hour, or is in hot weather, consider a sports drink. "I recommend staying away from the stuff with 9,000 ingredients," says Casa. "You just need the essentials—fluid, carbohydrates, and electrolytes."

TRY AND TRY AGAIN: The only way to determine which drinks work for you is by testing them. "Some products may not taste good to you, while others may sit in your stomach in a bad way," says Casa. If you're the type of salty sweater who finds white streaks on your jersey after a ride, you may need a drink with more sodium. For extreme salt sweaters, Casa suggests adding $1/4$ teaspoon of salt to 16 ounces of sports drink (that's 600 mg of sodium). If you find that a sports drink upsets your stomach, try diluting it with water. "Just never start a big event with a new product in your bottle," says Casa. "That's a recipe for disaster."

The Caffeine Question

Caffeine may be the most widely used stimulant drug in the world, especially among cyclists. From roadies who sip espresso to downhillers who pound an energy drink before a race, the allure of a preride pick-me-up transcends cycling's cultural differences. The jolt is very real. Caffeine is an endurance performance booster, says sports nutrition researcher Stacy Sims, PhD. "It increases your power output and time to exhaustion, and lowers your perceived exertion." In other words, you'll pedal longer, more powerfully, and feel less tired.

HOW IT WORKS

During endurance efforts, caffeine helps the body use fat as fuel, so you don't burn through your carbohydrate stores as quickly, says Sims. A preride cappuccino could improve your town line sprint as well. "Caffeine increases the calcium content of muscle, which enhances the strength of the muscle contraction," she says—good news for riders looking to hammer big gears. The performance boost you get from caffeine is also a result of how it hot-wires your central nervous system, says Matthew Ganio, PhD, director of the human performance laboratory at the University of Arkansas. "Caffeine crowds out a calming brain chemical called adenosine," he says. You become more alert, you react faster, and you don't feel like you're working as hard, all of which add up to training or competing at a higher intensity for a longer period of time and being more agile in a pack.

WHAT YOU NEED

It takes about 3 to 6 milligrams of caffeine per kilogram of body weight (190 to 380 mg for a

140-pound rider) for most people to notice a performance benefit, says Mindy Millard-Stafford, PhD, director of the exercise physiology laboratory at Georgia Tech in Atlanta. "Higher doses are more likely to cause side effects," she says, "and there's no evidence that extra caffeine provides additional performance benefits." During training, start at the lower end of the dose recommendation and work up to the level that's best for you.

WHERE TO GET IT

Although coffee is the most widely consumed caffeine source, you may get a bigger jolt from spiked gels, bars, supplements, or even gum. "Chemicals in coffee impair some of the pep that caffeine provides," says sports dietitian Molly Morgan, RD. "What's more, depending on the preparation method, brand, and variety, the caffeine content in java can vary greatly." Packaged sports nutrition products, with caffeine amounts printed on the label, are more accurate sources.

FIVE STIMULATING TRUTHS ABOUT CAFFEINE

1. It Will Not Dehydrate You

"In reasonable doses, caffeine alone won't lead to more bathroom breaks during a ride or a greater risk of dehydration," says Millard-Stafford. The upshot, she says, is that regardless of whether you supplement with caffeine, you don't need additional fluid to avoid performance-sapping dehydration during a ride. The long-held belief that caffeine can muck with your body's ability to regulate heat during exercise in hot weather has also been muted by science.

2. It Affects Everyone Differently

Before breaking out a venti on event day, Ganio suggests testing what caffeine does to you during hard training sessions. "If you feel jittery, anxious, or notice your heart racing, dial back the amount you take in before a ride," says Ganio. "If you can't find a caffeine level that leaves you feeling comfortable, skip it. Side effects can impair performance."

3. You Can Develop a Tolerance

Your body eventually adapts to the effects of caffeine, limiting the performance benefit. If you regularly drink more than five daily cups of coffee, Ganio recommends tapering your intake by half a cup per day for several days before a big ride. Save higher amounts of caffeine for before and during actual events.

4. Timing Is Everything

It takes 60 minutes for caffeine to start affecting the body, so imbibe 1 hour before a ride. "For rides lasting 2 hours or more, take half of your caffeine before and the other half in divided amounts during the ride," says Ganio, "making sure to consume the remainder when there is more than an hour left in your ride."

Say you plan to take 200 mg of caffeine for a 3-hour ride: Aim for 100 mg 1 hour before you get on the bike, and 50 mg at the beginning of each hour thereafter.

5. Training Trumps It

"While caffeine can boost performance by 3 to 5 percent, training can bring about improvements by upwards of 50 percent," Ganio says. There's also the possibility of getting over-amped and going out too hard too soon, leaving you with nothing in the tank well before the ride's end. Bottom line: No amount of caffeine will turn a donkey into a thoroughbred.

Race or Event Nutrition

The 24 hours before a big event are a special occasion. You're going to be blowing through a lot of energy on your ride, and you need to stock your body with the carbs and protein it needs to help you ride strong. It's one of those rare times when you'll want to eat more than your typical amount of daily calories. Enjoy yourself, but for peak performance pay special attention to the foods you're choosing. Drinking enough fluids is also vital to your performance.

THE DAY BEFORE

Losing as little as 2 percent of your body weight due to dehydration can lead to a 10 percent drop in athletic performance. Because the majority of Americans, including athletes, are chronically dehydrated, you may be 2 percent dehydrated before you even start working out. So focusing on fluids is vital. Throughout the day before a big event, drink around 96 to 128 ounces of fluid, or 12 to 16 eight-ounce glasses. It may seem like a lot, but when you spread it across meals and snacks, it's easily achievable and will help you feel ready to ride. Start first thing. When you get out of bed, drink 16 to 20 ounces of water; it's a simple way to jumpstart your hydration for today or any day. With meals, drink at least 20 ounces of water, and between meals drink another 16 to 20 ounces. By lunch, you'll already have about 60 ounces down the hatch.

Breakfast should be rich in carbohydrates and contain moderate amounts of protein and fat. This means oatmeal, granola, or whole wheat pancakes for carbs and eggs, yogurt, or maybe tofu for protein. Skip the breakfast meats. They're typically higher in saturated fat and sodium, and we're looking for "cleaner" sources of energy in this crucial time period.

As for between-meal snacks, they're a good way to moderately increase the amount of carbs you consume the day before a big event without going through the sometimes disruptive process of carbo-loading. (If you're experienced with carbo-loading, you're welcome to do it, but now is not the time to experiment.) Again, think clean sources of carbohydrate and protein, like whole grain bread and peanut butter, yogurt and granola, hummus with cut vegetables, or an energy bar with balanced carbs and protein. Repeat with a similar snack between lunch and dinner.

Speaking of lunch, skip the all-you-can-eat Indian buffet and have a sandwich, which lets you build your own meal of high-quality carbohydrates and protein. Make it a big one: This is your opportunity to chow down on thick slices of multigrain bread, lean turkey breast, firm tofu or hummus, and plenty of fresh veggies. Add a salad and a side of rice, pasta, or potatoes or extra carbs that are easy on the stomach.

THE NIGHT BEFORE

While a lot of people automatically go for the heaping bowl of pasta for dinner the night before a race, a meal that's rich in carbohydrates but not overloaded with them gets the job done and is less likely to sit heavily in your gut all night. Grilled fish served on a bed of brown rice with a big salad and baked potato works very well. Eat until you're satisfied, but there's no benefit in gorging yourself. Continue consuming fluids throughout the evening and save the booze for after your ride.

IN THE MORNING

This is where your tried-and-true habits take precedence over science. Lance Armstrong was a cornflake guy. He liked them and found he rode well after eating them, so he always started his breakfast there and often moved on to an omelet and some risotto afterward for some satisfying protein and complex carbs. You want to replenish the carbohydrate stores you burned while you slept, but it's important to eat foods you know will treat you well when you start riding. Two to three hours before the start, eat what you like, aim for some complex carbs and protein, and skip heavy foods like breakfast meats or dairy if you know they don't agree with you before a ride.

TOP OFF THE TANK

In the hours between your final pre-event meal and the main event, have a bottle of

60

Percent increase in postexercise muscle repair among study subjects who ate protein right after working out, compared with when they ingested it over 3.5 hours, according to *The American Journal of Clinical Nutrition.* Good protein sources include hard-boiled eggs, milk, or a turkey sandwich.

BETTER RECOVERY MEANS BETTER TRAINING

DON'T HANDICAP YOUR TRAINING BY NEGLECTING POSTWORKOUT recovery nutrition. Immediately after you get off your bike, while you're stretching, drink a carbohydrate-rich recovery drink or a shake that's mostly carbs with a little protein. Within an hour, sit down to a meal with carbs from whole grains and/or fresh vegetables and lean protein from chicken, turkey, fish, or tofu. Keep consuming fluids throughout the rest of the day.

Good examples of postworkout meals include:

➤ Grilled salmon on buckwheat noodles, green salad, and roasted veggies

➤ Stir-fry with teriyaki-marinated tofu, mixed veggies, and brown rice

➤ Spinach salad with roasted chicken, walnuts, sliced pears, a little crumbled blue cheese, and balsamic vinaigrette

➤ Sushi (My favorite for after a big training ride is a sashimi platter, brown rice, and a seaweed salad.)

sports drink in order to continue hydrating and topping off your carbohydrate stores. Have an energy bar or light carbohydrate snack available in case you feel a hunger pang in the hour before the start.

Fueling on the Bike

If you want to ride strong and get the most out of your training, you have to stay nourished. First rule? Eat *before* you ride. Too many cyclists skimp on fuel before their rides, which prevents them from getting the maximum training benefit from the workouts. "It's important to have good glycogen stores to begin with," says San Millán. That's because when these stores are low, the body breaks down muscle protein for fuel. "In a way, the muscles are actually eating themselves to feed themselves," he says. Ride hungry too often, and you'll end up overtrained: When exercise-stressed muscles routinely don't get fuel when they need it, they grow weaker, not stronger.

Once you're rolling, scheduling your carbs is as important as choosing them. Use this handy guide to figure out what you need to eat when.

Timing Matters

YOUR RIDE	EAT THIS	WHEN
An easy and short ride (45 to 90 minutes)	1 banana + 2 fig bars (**OR** nothing, if you've eaten within the last 3 hours.)	**As you're kitting up**
An easy but long ride (2+ hours). You'll be burning mostly fat, but you still need energy for the long haul. You want foods that digest at different rates for quick energy, plus slower-digesting items that will keep you rolling beyond the 90-minute mark.	1 cup yogurt + granola **OR** 1 English muffin + nut butter	**About 30 minutes before you roll**
Moderate to tempo pace; a short ride (45 to 90 minutes with some climbs and/or harder efforts). As intensity rises, so do your carb needs. Digestion also slows because your blood is fueling your muscles rather than your gut. Choose easily digestible carbs (lower in fiber) with a little protein.	1 turkey sandwich **OR** 1 cup cereal + low-fat milk + berries	**About 2 hours before you start pedaling.** You want enough time to digest, but not so much that you feel hungry before you start.
Moderate to tempo; a long ride (2+ hours with some climbs and/or harder efforts). You'll be out there working for a pretty long time, so you want to start with a fairly full tank.	1 bagel + nut butter + honey **OR** 1 bowl oatmeal + raisins	**About 2 hours preride.** Also take food with you.
A hard* and short ride (45 to 90 minutes; cyclocross practice, intervals). You're going to suck your glycogen stores dry, so start on full to avoid hitting the wall before you're done. Digestion will also be compromised, so you don't want to eat anything that'll come back up. This means not too much fat, which slows stomach emptying.	Pancakes or waffles + nuts + fruit	**About 2½ to 3 hours before you ride.** You want plenty of time for your food to digest. About 15 minutes before you start, top your tank with 100 calories of something easy to digest, such as a few sport chews, half an energy bar, fig bars, or sports drink.
A hard* and long ride (2+ hours; an epic beatdown of any variety). You'll need carbs, and plenty of them. Start by eating 400 to 600 calories, about 60 percent of them carbohydrates.	Tortilla + eggs + cooked veggies + potatoes	**About 3 to 4 hours preride.** You'll be eating a lot of food and you want plenty of time to digest. About 30 minutes before go time, top your tank with 100–200 calories of something easy to digest such as sport chews, an energy bar, fig bars, or sports drink.

*Within an hour after a hard effort, restock your fuel tank with a snack or meal that provides 250 to 300 calories' worth of carbs.

The final key to keeping your engine revved is remembering to *use* the above information. On long rides, it's easy to lose track of how much time has passed since you last ate or drank. One easy solution: Set a timer on your watch, smartphone, or bike computer to go off at regular intervals. This can remind you to hydrate and fuel up as well as help train you to reach for your bottle or snack more regularly. Set your timer based on the following guidelines:

- On average, you should steadily drink 4 to 6 ounces of water or sports drink (which can also help replenish carbohydrates) every 10 to 15 minutes.

- Eat 7 to 10 grams of carbs every 15 to 20 minutes after you've ridden 45 minutes. Choose high-carb, low-fat snacks: a date (7 grams of carbs), half a banana (14 g), or half of a gel packet (6 g).

CHAPTER 5

Strength Training

Machines don't break records. Muscles do.

—Lon Haldeman, US ultra-distance road racer

BUILDING SPEED AND ENDURANCE ON THE BIKE IS ABOUT MORE than how many miles you pedal. "You also need total-body strength, power, core stability, and flexibility," says Greg Moore, a performance specialist at St. Vincent Sports Performance in Indianapolis. Lifting weights can train your riding muscles to last longer and work harder. When you do sport-specific exercises such as squats and leg presses for 8 to 12 weeks in the off-season, the muscle fibers you use for short, hard efforts become more resistant to fatigue, according to a report published in the *Scandinavian Journal of Medicine and Science in Sports.* Your brain also becomes more adept at recruiting the muscles you need to keep riding.

Below are more exercises than you will ever need, organized by macrocycle and then body part. During your base period, strength train 3 days a week, *at least* one exercise for each important area of the body: legs, glutes, core, and arms. For road cyclists, this period will typically be October through February. When you build (for roadies, usually March and April), lighten your load by doing the prescribed routine below, which focuses on high-intensity moves, twice a week. To maintain strength, we've also supplied you with maintenance exercises you should do twice a week during your race season. And for those of you short on time or without access to a gym, the chapter wraps up with an effective at-home routine.

Warm-Up

If you work at a desk and your main form of exercise is riding, you should carefully consider your approach to weight work, says fitness expert Peter Park, founder of Platinum Fitness in Summerland, California. White-collar cyclists already spend hours hunched forward and should avoid activities that reinforce that position, like crunches and bench presses. "They make the pattern worse, because you're making yourself into a ball," Park says.

Instead, focus on mobility and active stretching—activities that will reverse posture problems by opening up your body and allowing you to do weight work safely and properly. "I always tell my clients, 'You have to earn the right to lift,'" Park says. These moves make an ideal warm-up.

The Founder

With feet shoulder-width apart, bend your knees slightly and pull your hips behind you, keeping your weight on your heels. Expand your chest, keeping arms back and shoulders pulling down toward your butt. Lift your arms in front of you as high as you can.

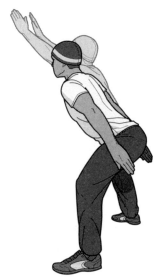

The Lunge Stretch

Do a lunge, front leg slightly bent, back foot facing forward and back heel pressing down. Extend your spine at the hips and raise your arms. You should feel a stretch in the hip flexors of the back leg. Laterally flex your body away from the back leg. Hold for 20 seconds per leg.

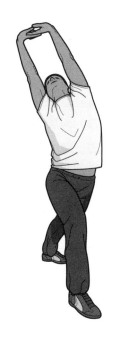

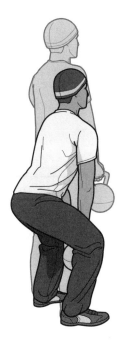

The Wall Squat

Stand facing a wall (to keep your form in check) with a 6-inch gap between your toes and the wall. Hold a kettlebell or dumbbell in both hands. Keeping your chest expanded and your back tight, squat by pushing your hips back before bending your knees. Keep your weight on your heels, with feet shoulder-width apart and toes out. Lower to a sitting position. As you stand, engage your glutes, lower back, and quads. Near the top of the movement, push your hips forward to accentuate glute and quad contraction.

During Base Work

LEGS

Admit it: You want legs that can power you to the town line sprint podium. But it wouldn't hurt if they were also the envy of your entire Sunday morning club ride. The key to achieving distinct muscle definition, says Sam Iannetta, a certified trainer and owner of Functional Fitness Wellness Centers in Boulder, Colorado, is to trade heavy weights for lighter ones and do more repetitions.

These moves work your legs from every angle for optimal shaping, not to mention balanced strength and stability. Do them 3 nonconsecutive days a week, aiming for two or three sets of 18 to 20 reps. Choose a weight that's challenging but light enough so you can maintain form until the last few reps, at which point your muscles should feel fatigued.

Bulgarian Squat

Grab a pair of dumbbells and stand with your back to a chair or bench. Extend your right leg backward, placing the top of your foot on the chair. Bend your left leg until your thigh is almost parallel to the floor. Press back to the starting position. Repeat for a full set, then switch legs.

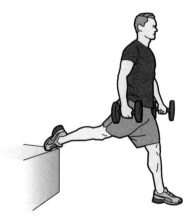 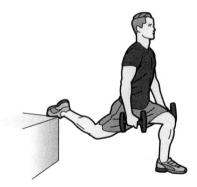

Single-Leg Step Down

Hold a dumbbell in each hand and stand with your right foot on a 6- to 12-inch-high step, allowing your left leg to dangle. Keeping your chest lifted and back straight, slowly lower your left foot as though dipping your toe into water, without touching the floor. Then straighten your right leg and rise onto the ball of your foot. Return to start and repeat for a full set, then switch legs.

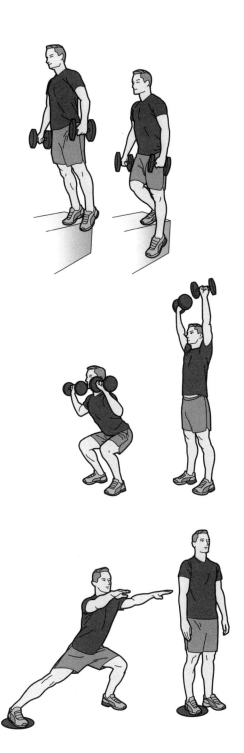

Dumbbell Squat to Overhead Press

Stand with your feet shoulder-width apart. Hold dumbbells at your shoulders, palms facing forward. Lower into a squat until your thighs are nearly parallel to the floor. Quickly return to standing and immediately press both dumbbells overhead. Return to start.

Slider Squat

Stand with a slider (or paper plate) underneath your right foot, arms down at your sides. Lift your arms straight out in front of you and lower into a squat while sliding your right foot to the side until your left thigh is parallel to the floor. Straighten your left leg, pull the right leg back to start, and lower your arms. Finish the set, then switch sides.

TURN YOUR CRANKS FASTER

A STUDY IN THE *EUROPEAN JOURNAL OF APPLIED PHYSIOLOGY* found that 3 weeks of thrice-weekly strength training sessions for the knee extensors (i.e., quads) improved torque—the force that rotates the cranks—by 17 percent among master cyclists (ages 35 plus) and 6 percent in a similar group in their mid-20s. The masters also saw improvements in their cycling efficiency—a bonus because with age comes muscle loss, which robs endurance.

KNEE EXTENSIONS

ON A LEG-EXTENSION MACHINE, SELECT A WEIGHT you can lift no more than 10 times. With your ankles behind the pads, extend your legs, then lower. Repeat for three sets of 10.

Stability Ball Hamstring Curl

Lie on your back with your feet on a stability ball. Inhale, tightening your abs, back, and butt muscles. Lift up off the floor to create a straight line from feet to shoulders. Exhale and bend your knees, using your heels to pull the ball toward your butt (feet will be flat on the ball). Return to the starting position. Do 10 to 15 repetitions. Rest for 30 seconds, then repeat. When you can do two sets of 15, add a third set.

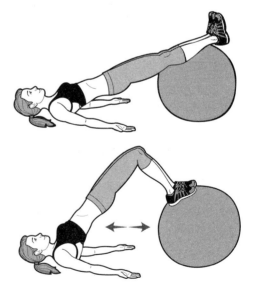

GLUTES

Strengthening your upper-outer glutes can improve your pedaling power and reduce pain in your knees, hips, and lower back—without activating overworked hip flexor muscles, according to the *Journal of Orthopaedic and Sports Physical Therapy*. Do these moves three times a week.

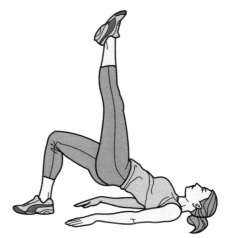

Single-Leg Bridge

Lie on your back with your left leg raised, your right foot flat on the floor, and arms at your sides. Contract your glutes and raise your hips until your body forms a straight line from your right knee to your shoulders. Pause, then lower to start. Do 10 to 12 reps per side.

IS LIFTING HEAVY WEIGHTS THE BEST WAY TO BUILD MUSCLE?

IT'S ACTUALLY THE FASTEST WAY TO BUILD overall (or maximal) strength, which leads to higher levels of muscular efficiency, agility, and mobility. But if you want low-intensity endurance strength without the bulk, you're better off lightening the load. "When cyclists push on the pedals, the force they exert is a small percentage of their maximal strength (1 to 3 percent on flat terrain at 100 rpm)," says Stuart Phillips, PhD, kinesiology professor at McMaster University in Hamilton, Ontario. Even climbing uses well below the maximum. You'll gain the same amount of lean muscle lifting three sets, each to fatigue, of lighter weights (10 to 15 pounds) as you would lifting heavier weights (25 to 30 pounds).

Source: *Journal of Applied Physiology*

Side Step

Tie an exercise band above your knees and stand with your legs hip-width apart. Take a big step to the right with your right foot, then a small step in that direction with your left foot, returning them to hip-width and keeping the band taut. Do five to six reps on each side.

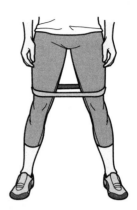

Clam

Tie an exercise band around your lower thighs and lie on your left side, knees bent. Rest your right hand on the floor and your left arm under your head. Keeping your heels together, lift your right knee as far as you can, then lower it. Do 10 to 12 reps per side.

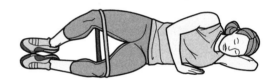

MUSCLE MEAT

IF YOU FIND IT MORE DIFFICULT WITH each birthday to maintain lean muscle mass, help yourself to a bigger cut of steak. A study published in *Applied Physiology, Nutrition, and Metabolism* concluded that, of 35 male test subjects whose average age was 59, those who ate 6 ounces of beef before a resistance-training workout gained more muscle than those who ate less. For best results, treat yourself after your workout. "That's when muscles are most receptive to the amino acids in protein," says Phillips, the senior study author. But, he says, there is no added benefit associated with more meat: "Other studies have found that 12 ounces isn't better than 6."

CORE

If you're not doing core work, you should be. Research on cyclists shows that when core muscles fatigue, pedaling mechanics break down, paving the way for poor performance and injury. No time, you say? That's no excuse. You need only 4 minutes to hone your core, says Allison Westfahl, an exercise physiologist in Boulder, Colorado. Here she details the moves she prescribes for pro clients like Team Garmin-Sharp's Tom Danielson. Perform one set of each exercise, resting 15 seconds between moves. Aim for three sessions a week. If you can, tack the routine onto the end of a ride. A study in the *Journal of Strength and Conditioning Research* reported that cyclists who cooled down with a core workout had significantly better lactate clearance, which helps reduce muscle fatigue, than those who did nothing.

Prone Snow Angels

Lie facedown, arms extended along your sides. Gently squeeze your glutes and slowly raise your feet, chest, and hands no more than 6 inches off the floor. Sweep your arms overhead and separate your feet. Try to touch your hands above your head. Return to the start position, relaxing your feet, chest, and arms. Do 15 reps.

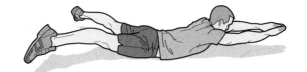

Mountain Climbers

Start in a pushup position with a small towel or paper plate under each foot. Squeeze your shoulder blades together and pull your lower abs toward your spine. Without rocking or swaying your hips, slowly slide your right knee toward your chest, then slowly push it back. Repeat with the left knee. That's 1 rep; do 15.

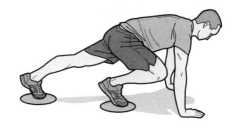

Seated Boat with Isometric Side Push

Sit on the floor, knees bent and heels lightly touching the floor. Make a fist with your left hand and press it into your right palm about 6 inches in front of your chest. Keeping your legs steady, twist your torso to the right. Hold, pushing your left fist into your right palm for 15 seconds. Twist to the left and repeat.

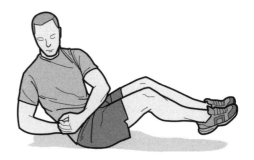

Plank with Alternating Knee Drops

Get into a pushup position with your forearms on the floor, elbows underneath your shoulders, and feet 8 to 10 inches apart. Your body should form a straight diagonal line. Slowly drop your right knee to the floor, then return to the start position. Drop the left knee. That's 1 rep; complete 15.

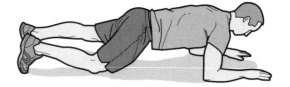

GET A JUMP ON THE COMPETITION

EVERY MUSCLE IN YOUR BODY CONSISTS OF thousands of fibers bundled in units that are activated by the brain. The more units you can engage, the more power your brain can call on during hard efforts. Explosive jumping exercises such as plyometrics not only train your neuromuscular pathways but also teach your body to adapt to high-speed movements without wasting energy, so more power goes into your pedals. Researchers have found that just 1 month of plyometric training twice a week can increase your power endurance by 17 percent. This means you'll be stomping out longer sprints and charging up hills in your big ring. After you have a few weeks of general training under your belt, do squat jumps twice a week.

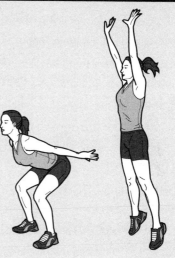

SQUAT JUMPS: Stand with feet shoulder-width apart, arms at sides. Sit into a squat, lowering until your thighs are parallel to the floor. Jump up explosively and reach for the ceiling. Land gently and lower into another squat. Do two sets of 10.

ARMS

Most of the attention in cycling is focused on your legs and lungs, understandably. Strong arms can also play a critical role in on-bike performance—most important, by fighting off fatigue. "Having stronger biceps and triceps means your arms will be under less metabolic stress as you ride," says Iñigo San Millán, PhD, director of the Human Performance Laboratory at the University of Colorado's Anschutz Health and Wellness Center in Denver. "Those muscles can then help remove lactate from your system during the ride, instead of producing it." That means more energy on long rides and more power for climbs. The key to efficiency, says San Millán, is to add strength without bulk. Try three sets of 12 to 15 repetitions of the following exercises two to three times a week, using dumbbells that total about 75 percent of the maximum weight that you can comfortably manage.

Hammer Curl

Stand straight, a dumbbell in each hand, palms facing your sides. Keeping upper arms tight against your body, raise the dumbbells until your forearms are nearly vertical and your thumbs face your shoulders. Slowly lower to original position.

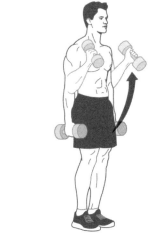

Lying Triceps Extension

Lie on your back on the floor, knees bent, feet flat. Hold a dumbbell in each hand, palms facing in, arms at your sides. Extend your arms toward the ceiling and slowly bend your elbows, lowering the dumbbells until they're at either side of your head. Repeat by raising arms toward the ceiling again, not by lowering them back to the floor as they were at the start.

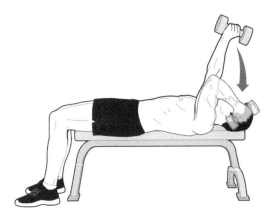

Military Pushup

Assume the pushup position. Tighten your abs and glutes to keep your back in a straight line. Slowly lower yourself to the floor, keeping your elbows against your body and in line with your shoulders. Push back up to return to the starting position.

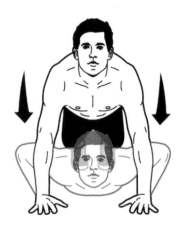

During Build

TRAIN YOUR MUSCLES TO FIRE FAST

Strength training is an off-season must for cyclists. Here's the catch: Weight lifting teaches your muscles to produce power at slow speed. Sure, you'll start the season stronger, but unless you teach those newly formed fibers to fire like lightning, you won't be faster. High-velocity pedaling power takes high-energy, high-repetition moves to train your muscles to detonate on demand.

To turn all your hard work in the gym into cycling-specific strength, do this routine twice a week for 4 weeks on nonconsecutive days. Perform two or three sets, or until you can no longer perform the moves quickly with good form. Rest 2 to 3 minutes between sets. Finish each session with 10 minutes of low-resistance, high-rpm spinning on your bike or trainer to flush out your legs and train your muscles to continue firing fast while fatigued.

High Step

Stand facing a box that is knee high. Plant your right foot on the box so your left leg is extended behind you with only your toes on the ground. Raise your arms in front of you for balance or place your hands on your hips. Keeping your right foot planted, step up on your right leg, touch the box briefly with your left foot, and lower your body back to start, keeping your right foot on the box. Repeat for a set, then switch sides. Aim for a cadence of one rep per second, or faster if you can do it without losing form. Do 15 to 20 reps per leg.

Jack Squats

Stand with your feet hip- to shoulder-width apart, arms at sides. While raising your arms straight out in front of you, bend your knees and hips until your thighs are parallel to the floor. Return to start. Do 30 reps.

Lunge Jumps

Stand with your right leg forward and your left leg extended behind you. Bend your right knee and dip your left knee toward the floor, so you're in a lunge position. With arms straight out in front of you, swiftly jump up and switch legs in the air, landing in the opposite position. When your back knee touches the ground, jump again. Do 12 to 15 reps.

Applause Pushup

Lie facedown on an exercise ball with both hands on the floor. Walk your hands out until they're directly below your shoulders and the ball is under your legs (under thighs is easiest; shins is hardest). Keeping your torso straight, bend your elbows and lower your chest toward the floor until your arms are bent 90 degrees. Push up as hard as you can, clap your hands once, and return to the starting position before immediately dropping into another repetition. These are tough. Start with a few and work up to 10 to 15 reps.

During Peak Muscle Maintenance

Your legs, butt, and arms get nonstop use—and sometimes abuse—as you're cranking down the road or trail. But you neglect three important muscle groups when you ride. It's too bad, because keeping these forgotten muscles strong could improve your cycling. Do the following exercises twice a week when you're in season.

Abdominals

Strong abs help transfer power from our arms pulling on the bar to our legs pushing the pedals. You climb better and sprint harder when your abs are peachy. Here's one of the best abdominal exercises, according to a study from the American Council on Exercise.

Lie face-up on the floor, lower back pressed to the ground, hands cupping your ears. Bring knees to a 45-degree angle and slowly make a pedaling motion. Alternately touch your left elbow to your right knee, then your right elbow to your left knee. Do 10 to 12 reps.

Lumbar Muscles

These lower back muscles go unused while we ride, so they're weak and susceptible to fatigue and cramping. This exercise will keep them strong and improve your balance:

Get on your hands and knees, with your back straight and head and neck in line with your spine. Slowly raise your right arm and left leg, bringing them in line with your back so your fingers are pointing straight ahead and your toes are pointing back. Hold, then lower and repeat with the other arm and leg. Do 10 to 12 reps on each side.

Trapezius

Strengthening your trapezius, the muscle that runs between your shoulders and up along your neck, helps keep your upper torso strong to support you on the long haul without neck pain problems. These shrugs can help.

Stand with feet apart, holding a dumbbell in each hand, palms facing your thighs. Raise your shoulders straight up toward your ears. Hold, then slowly lower. Do 10 to 12 reps.

Home Body

Getting to and from the gym can be a major time suck, especially when you'd rather be riding. But with the right equipment plus a few key moves, you can get stronger at home—and have more time for the bike. Here's your guide.

ESSENTIAL TOOLS

Dumbbells

Simple and versatile, you can use a set of dumbbells to work nearly every muscle in your body.

LOOK FOR: A range of 5 to 25 pounds

Stability Ball

Best known as a core-sculpting tool, it can also double as a bench.

LOOK FOR: One that's burst resistant

Plyo Box or Step

Use for step-ups and plyometric moves that build leg strength and power.

LOOK FOR: A nonslip platform and adjustable height

Resistance Bands

Add challenge to lower-body moves. Also good for stretching pedal-weary legs.

LOOK FOR: A set with a variety of resistance levels

Sliding Discs

Slip these under your feet or hands to make muscles work harder with every move.

LOOK FOR: Discs that work on your surface of choice, whether floor or carpet

All-In-One Tool

This workout gear can be adapted for multiple types of exercises, which makes total-body training a snap.

LOOK FOR: The TRX Home Kit suspension trainer. Attach it almost anywhere for a head-to-toe workout ($200).

The Workout

Five at-home moves to power up your ride. Do three sets of 12 reps.

Dumbbell T

WORKS UPPER BACK, GLUTES

Grab an 8- to 10-pound dumbbell in each hand and stand with your feet slightly more than shoulder-width apart, arms down in front of you. Lower into a squat, keeping your knees behind your toes. Raise the dumbbells out to your sides until they're at shoulder level, then lower.

Double Leg Curl

WORKS CORE, GLUTES, HAMSTRINGS

Lie on the floor with your heels on top of a stability ball and your arms extended out to the sides at shoulder level. Lift your hips until you form a diagonal line from heels to shoulders. Bend your knees, pulling the ball toward your butt. Return to start.

Step-Up

WORKS HIPS, GLUTES, QUADS

Stand facing a box or step. Place your right foot on the box, then lift your left knee to hip level in front of you. Step down with your left leg, then the right. Repeat. Complete the prescribed number of reps, then switch legs.

Sliding Lunge

WORKS GLUTES, INNER THIGHS, QUADS, HAMSTRINGS

Stand with your feet hip-width apart, left foot on top of a sliding disc, hands in front of you. Bend your right knee and push your hips back as you slide your left leg out to the side. Return to start. Do all the reps, then switch legs.

Hamstring Stretch

WORKS GLUTES, HAMSTRINGS

Lie face-up on the floor. Grab the end of a resistance band in each hand and loop it around your right foot. Extend your right leg toward the ceiling and hold it there for 5 seconds, gently pulling the leg toward you. Return to start. Complete all the reps, then switch legs.

CHAPTER 6

Flexibility

Doctors can tell if they're operating on a cyclist just by looking at the internal tissues—they're strong and flexible, there's more muscle and less fat.

—Thomas Dickson, MD, cycling physician

SCOTT HOLZ BELIEVES IN STRETCHING—AND NOT JUST because he personally benefits from greater flexibility. As a bike-fit expert and global manager of Specialized Bicycle Component University, Holz has worked with such ProTour riders as Fabian Cancellara and has seen the way pliant muscles help even the world's best cyclists find room to improve. "Flexibility is one of the biggest limiting factors for achieving your most powerful bike position," Holz says.

The upside of having supple muscles is huge: The more flexible you are, the more aerodynamic you can become—which helps you go faster with less effort. Regular stretching also quiets aches and strains that can limit your mileage, speeds the replenishment of glycogen stores in your muscles, and helps counteract the effects of aging, which causes muscles to lose elasticity.

The key is to know what to do and when. Research shows that stretching before exertion can weaken muscles. Instead, try some dynamic stretches. They increase a joint's range of motion through progressive movements, promote blood flow to muscles, and fire up your neuromuscular system. Dynamic stretches may also improve power and general flexibility, says Malachy McHugh, PhD, director of research at the Nicholas Institute of Sports Medicine and Athletic Trauma in New York City. On the bike, stretch dynamically by spinning easy for a few minutes then putting your legs through increasingly exaggerated movements—dropping your heels to stretch your calves and getting out of the saddle to move your hips front and back, side to side.

Save the static stretching for after your ride, when your muscles are warm (or later, after a hot shower). To figure out where you're tightest, take the test below. Once you identify problem areas, get to work on them—often. "Consistency is important," says Holz. "You're better off doing 10 to 15 minutes 4 days a week than an hour once a week." That's because gaining flexibility is a long-term process, says Andy Pruitt, EdD, founder of the Boulder Center for Sports Medicine in Colorado. "It takes 6 weeks to achieve a true length change in muscle or tendon structure," he says.

The Bicycling Flexibility Test

ILIOTIBIAL BAND, QUADS, HIP FLEXORS

THE TEST: Lie on a table or high bench and let half of your thighs extend off the edge. Dangle one foot and bend the other knee, pulling it toward your chest until your lower back touches the bench. Have a partner observe what happens.

. . . If your dangling knee falls to the side rather than forming a straight line from the hip, your iliotibial band, which runs along the thigh to the calves, is tight.

WHY IT MATTERS: The iliotibial band stabilizes the knee. If it's tight, it can rub against the knee and become inflamed, an overuse injury known as iliotibial band friction syndrome.

THE FIX: Leg roll

Lie on your side, your thigh resting on a foam roller. Ease your leg along the cylinder, using your weight to apply pressure to the tissue. Roll up and down the band for 60 seconds, then repeat on the other leg. Spend extra time on tender areas.

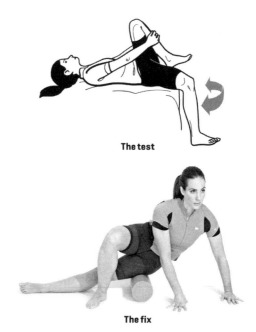

The test

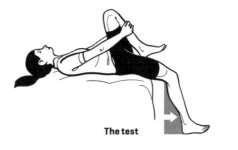

The fix

. . . If the ankle on your extended leg sticks out beyond your knee, you have tight quads. The straighter the extended leg, the tighter the muscles.

WHY IT MATTERS: Your quads produce power, and a limited range of motion prevents some muscle fibers from firing, says cycling coach Carson Christen, MS.

THE FIX: Lying quad stretch

Lie on your stomach with your knees hip-width apart. Reach one arm back and grasp the opposite ankle. Slowly pull the heel in toward your butt. Keep your pelvis flat on the floor. Hold for 20 seconds, then repeat on the other side.

The test

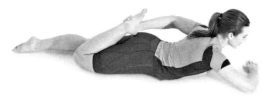

The fix

. . . If your extended thigh lifts so that the knee rises above your hip rather than remaining flat, your hip flexors aren't as flexible as they should be.

WHY IT MATTERS: The hip flexor muscles pull the leg up and over the top of the pedal stroke. Stretching them prevents lower back pain when you amp up your intensity.

THE FIX: Kneeling lunge

Kneel as shown below. Straighten your pelvis to align your pubic bone directly below your hip bones. Ease your hips down and forward, keeping your front knee directly over your ankle, and hold for 20 seconds. Repeat on the other side.

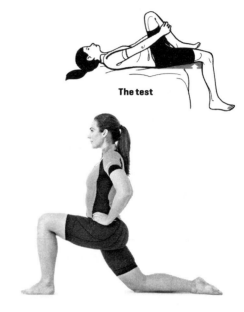

The test

The fix

GLUTES

THE TEST: Lie flat. Ask a partner to raise your leg as far as it can comfortably go, bending the knee. Estimate the angle your thigh forms to the floor: less than 90 degrees indicates tight glutes; 90 to 120 is typical. Test both legs.

WHY IT MATTERS: Tight glutes prevent you from achieving an aerodynamic position in the drops.

THE FIX: Pigeon pose

Kneel on the floor with one leg extended behind and the other bent at a 45-degree angle in front of you, ankle and knee touching the floor. Keeping your hips square, ease your pelvis toward the floor. Next, tilt forward and lower your chest toward the floor. Hold for 30 seconds, then repeat on the other side.

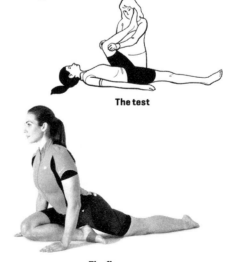

The test

The fix

HAMSTRINGS

THE TEST: Lie flat and have a partner raise one leg until your hamstring begins to tug. Estimate the angle formed with the floor: 55 degrees or less signals poor flexibility. Repeat with the other leg.

WHY IT MATTERS: Longer hamstrings let the pelvis tilt forward on the saddle, allowing for a more aero position. Plus, you'll get your glutes—the body's strongest muscles—more involved in pedaling.

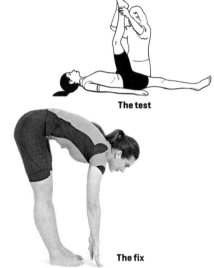

The test

THE FIX: Standing forward fold

Stand with feet hip-width apart and slowly bend at the waist, tilting your pelvis forward and keeping your back straight. Pause for 10 to 15 seconds when you feel a slight stretch in the back of your legs, then deepen the pose until you feel the hamstrings relax.

The fix

CALVES

THE TEST: Sit on a bench with your feet flat on the floor. Raise your toes while keeping your heels grounded. If you can't get your foot past 90 degrees, use the stretch at right.

WHY IT MATTERS: Tight calves and Achilles tendons force cyclists into an exaggerated, toe-down pedal stroke that transfers less power than a flatter foot. More flexible calves allow for a more powerful and efficient stroke—and also leave you less prone to cramping.

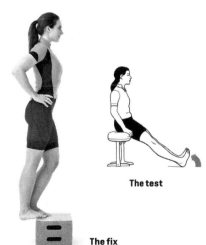

The test

THE FIX: Single heel drop stand, with the balls of your feet on a step

Lower one heel to stretch through the calf, ankle, and Achilles tendon. Hold for 10 seconds, then repeat a second time. Switch and stretch the other side.

The fix

Banish Back Pain

You expect sore quads, calves, and glutes after copious saddle time, but, according to a study in the *American Journal of Sports Medicine*, back pain is the most common overuse injury reported by competitive cyclists. Even if you don't pin on a race number every weekend, "simple yoga-based stretches align your spine; relieve back, neck, and shoulder pain; and create flexibility in your upper body," says Alyssa Dinowitz, founder of Athletes Yoga in Tempe, Arizona. Do this sequence two or three times a week to keep your back going strong.

Tilt and Hold

Sit up tall in a chair with your back straight and your feet flat on the floor. Bend your head and neck forward as far as possible, keeping your shoulders down. Lace your fingers together behind your head, elbows out to the sides, and press gently on the back of your head. Hold for eight deep breaths, then release. Repeat three times.

Spinal Twist

Sit on a mat and place your right foot on the floor outside your left knee. Slide your left foot back, tucking it under your right thigh. Inhale, lift your left arm overhead, then lower your elbow to the outside of your right knee. Place your right hand on the floor behind you; exhale and twist to the right. Hold for five breaths, then repeat on the other side.

Eagle Arm Pose

Stay seated and extend your arms in front of you at shoulder level. Cross your left arm over your right, raise your forearms perpendicular to the floor, and twist your palms inward until they touch. Inhale and raise your arms slightly; exhale and lower. That's one rep. Do five reps. Unwind, switch arms, and repeat.

Cat Cow

Start on all fours, back flat, eyes focused on the floor. Inhale. As you exhale, round your spine like a cat, drop your head, and tuck your chin toward your chest. Inhale, then arch your back toward the floor, lifting your hips, tailbone, and chest toward the ceiling, directing your gaze upward. Exhale as you return to cat pose. Do the sequence 10 times.

Unusual Stretches, Amazing Benefits

These five stretches will allow you to breathe easier, climb stronger, and pedal more fluidly in any position. Do them every day, and you'll ride better sooner.

Hip Flexor Stretch

Holding on to a wall or the back of a chair for balance, stand just in front of an exercise ball. Place your left instep on the ball and bend your right knee, extending your left leg back and pushing the ball away from you as you sink down into your hips as far as comfortably possible. Hold for 10 seconds. Return to standing position. Switch legs. Perform two to three times per leg.

CYCLING BENEFIT: Lengthens the hip flexor muscles on the front of your pelvis as well as those surrounding your groin for fuller, more powerful leg extension when you're out of the saddle.

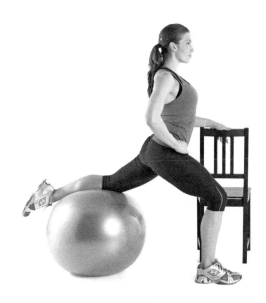

70

Percent less lower-back pain reported by study volunteers 3 months after they took a weekly yoga class for 16 weeks, according to the journal *Pain*.

Straddle-Seated Windmill

Sit tall with your legs extended and open wider than shoulder width. Extend your arms out to the sides at shoulder height. Twist to the left, reaching your right hand down to the outside of your left foot, while extending your left arm behind you. Hold for 10 seconds, return to the center, and switch sides. Perform two to three times per side.

CYCLING BENEFIT: Relieves lower-back tension and tightness, allowing for stronger, more complete power transfer from bar to pedals when jamming out of the saddle or pulling hard in a paceline.

Pro Tip

Stretching on the bike helps minimize fatigue. Coast, put your left foot down, then lean far to the right to stretch your back and your left leg. Then do the right leg.

SUPPLE MUSCLES AND ARTERIES

A STUDY PUBLISHED IN THE *AMERICAN JOURNAL OF PHYSIOLOGY–HEART AND CIRCULATORY PHYSIOLOGY* reports that there may be more to touching your toes than flexibility. It may also be a sign of how supple your cardiac arteries are. In a study of 526 adults, researchers found that subjects over the age of 40 who performed poorly on a sit-and-reach test also had stiffer arteries, which can lead to heart attacks. A separate study found that men and women who stretched for 13 weeks improved the pliability of their arteries by more than 20 percent. This is important for cyclists, who often neglect to stretch and aren't known for their great flexibility, but who also rely on healthy arteries to pedal down the road.

Thigh Lengthener

Kneel on a carpeted floor or mat with your knees hip-distance apart. Extend your arms in front of you, so they are straight out at shoulder height. Tuck your chin toward your chest and lean your body back as far as comfortably possible while maintaining a straight line from your shoulders to your knees. Hold 5 to 10 seconds. Contract abdominal and glute muscles to bring your body back to the starting position. Perform two to three times.

CYCLING BENEFIT: Loosens hips for smoother transitions in and out of the saddle when sprinting, accelerating, and climbing, and improves core strength and stability, which gives you a stronger platform to pedal against.

Chest Opener

Stand with your legs in a straddle stance. Place your hands behind your back on your hips and press your fingertips together. Slowly work your hands up your back as far as comfortable, pressing your palms together, if possible. Pivot your right foot and turn your body 90 degrees to the right. The back foot should rotate a little less, to provide better balance. Drop your shoulders and extend your chest, torso, and hips. Tilt your head slightly back to look up toward the ceiling. Hold for 10 seconds. Return to starting position and switch legs. Perform two times per side.

CYCLING BENEFIT: Opens chest and shoulder girdle to allow for maximum lung expansion while riding.

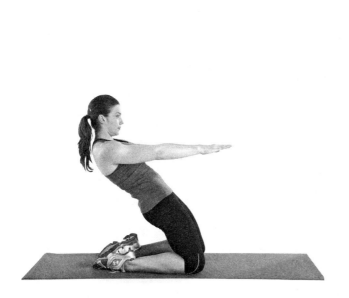

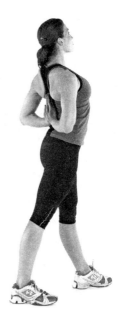

Shoulder Stand Scissors Kick

Lying on your back, pull your knees toward your chest and lift your hips and lower back off the floor. With your elbows on the floor, brace your hips with your hands. Extend your legs toward the ceiling. Keeping legs as straight as possible, scissor them, trying to lower them as close to the floor as comfortably possible. Hold for 5 seconds, then scissor your legs the opposite direction and repeat. Perform five to six times per leg.

CYCLING BENEFIT: Encourages blood flow back to the heart to revive tired, lactic acid–filled legs. Loosens hamstring, groin, and inner thigh muscles for maximum pedaling comfort.

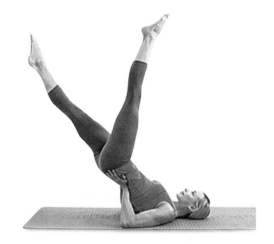

Roll Out the Kinks

The world would be a better place if all cyclists had the luxury of a daily post-ride massage. With a foam roller you can pretty much do the job yourself—minus the harp music. "As you roll a muscle back and forth on the dense foam cylinder, it breaks down adhesions and scar tissue," says Scott Levin, MD, sports medicine specialist at Somers Orthopaedic Surgery and Sports Medicine Group in New York. "It also warms and stretches muscles, increases circulation, and prevents soreness." Try this routine once or twice a day, 2 or 3 times a week. Roll back and forth slowly along the cylinder 10 to 12 times. Pause at tender spots, take a deep breath, and press your weight into them.

Hamstrings

Sit with your right leg on the roller, left knee bent, hands on the floor behind you. Roll from just above your knee to right below your glute. Switch legs.

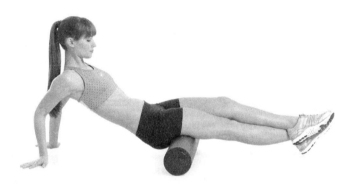

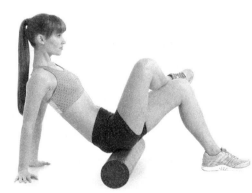

Glutes

Sitting on the roller, cross your right leg over your left knee and lean toward the right hip, hands on the floor for support. Roll the right cheek. Switch sides.

Quads

Lie facedown on the floor and place the roller under your hips. Lean on your right quad and roll between your hip and knee. Switch legs.

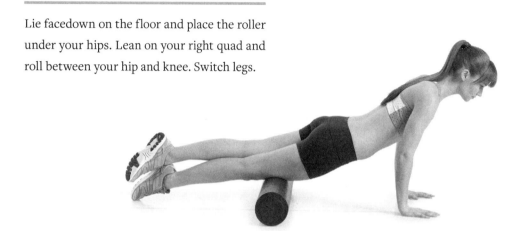

Back

Sit with the roller behind you. Lace your fingers behind your head and lean your upper back onto the roller. Tighten your abs and glutes and slowly roll up and down.

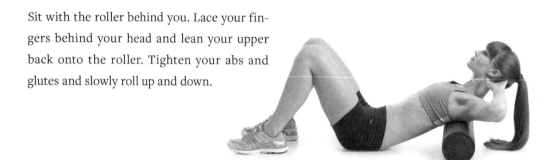

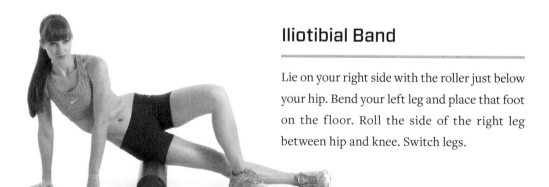

Iliotibial Band

Lie on your right side with the roller just below your hip. Bend your left leg and place that foot on the floor. Roll the side of the right leg between hip and knee. Switch legs.

Calves

Sit on the floor with your legs out, hands on the floor behind you. Place the roller under your knees. Roll along your calves from your knees to your ankles and back again.

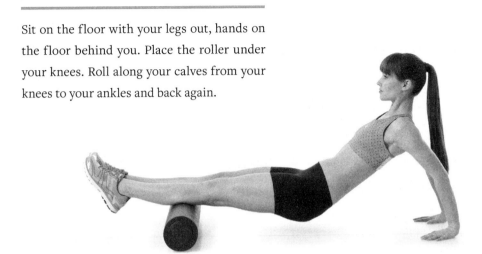

PART III

RIDE

Rev your metaphorical engines! It's time to get to the core of what it takes to cross the finish line of your first two-wheeled event. Whether your goal is to survive a multiday charity ride or ride 100 miles in one stretch, this section will break down the skills you'll need to master and the exact workouts you'll have to complete.

CHAPTER 7

Road Skills

There is no reason why a man on a smooth road should lose his balance on a bicycle; but he could.

—C. S. LEWIS, SCHOLAR, THEOLOGIAN, AND WRITER

NOW THAT YOU UNDERSTAND HOW TO PLAN AND EXECUTE A fitness-building training plan, it's time to address the other half of what makes a cyclist successful: bike-handling skills. Without them, your fitness can't shine. Take, for example, Team Boels-Dolmans rider Evelyn "Evie" Stevens. Her meteoric rise from amateur biker to professional cyclist is well-known, but what's not is the intense learning curve she had to overcome once she reached the top ranks. At the 2011 Giro Donne—the women's Tour of Italy—one of the stages included the 6,000-foot-high Passo di Mortirolo, a fearsome climb that should have suited her elite physiology.

Instead, Stevens told *Bicycling* magazine, "I crashed like every five minutes—I ate it. I kept racing but it was almost more frustrating. It was probably the lowest point in my cycling career." Stevens spent the next off-season in Boulder, Colorado, working on her bike-handling skills, and it paid off. She won the 2012 edition of the Fléche Wallonne, a prestigious race with a mountaintop finish.

Be like Evie. Improve your weaknesses and fine-tune your strengths. Become an efficient rider to maximize your fitness. Below are the tools you'll need.

Braking

Good bike riding is about efficiency. If you reduce waste through proper pedaling mechanics, body position, nutrition, gear selection, and even breathing, you will improve your overall performance on the road. One aspect of efficiency that's often overlooked is slowing down. By learning to brake skillfully, you can not only avoid accidents but also improve efficiency and save energy for the times when you need it. Here are some essential techniques.

FINGERS READY

Any time there's a wheel in front of you (i.e., you're drafting), rest your fingers on the brake levers. This way, you'll be able to brake quickly and minor slowdowns won't develop into emergency stop situations while your hands find the brakes.

KEEP IT EQUAL

In 99 percent of braking situations, you want to apply pressure evenly to each brake lever so that both tires share the load. This helps maintain stability and control. Practice on a grass field, sprinting up to speed, then slowing as fast as you can without skidding. You'll need to modulate finger pressure on each brake lever, much like antilock brakes on a car, to stop individual tires from skidding.

TURN SMART

Always brake before a turn. As you near the curve, apply equal pressure to the brakes to reach a manageable speed and then release the levers before you begin the turn to let your speed carry you through. Braking in a turn wreaks havoc on momentum, but if it's necessary for safety, use the rear brake only—remember "right rear" to keep them straight in your mind, unless you've reversed the cables—because a front-tire skid guarantees a crash. Skidding the rear may raise your heart rate, but it will allow you to steer out of trouble.

LEARN TO STOP HARD

When you master the emergency stop, you'll have greater overall stopping confidence because you'll know this move is there when you need it. For more braking power, put your hands in the drops. Then, for added stability, push your weight back behind the saddle by shifting your butt and straightening your arms. Practice on the grass, with the goal of not skidding. *Remember*: Fresh brake pads greatly increase stopping performance—replace them regularly. Consult with your bike shop if you're not sure when they are needed.

After you master these braking skills, you'll be able to anticipate, a key skill for every cyclist from beginner to Tour de France champion. When you anticipate that the rider in front of you is going to swerve, for example, you won't have to overreact by slamming on the brakes. In many scenarios, continuing to pedal while braking lightly will get you out of trouble. Plus, you won't be a yo-yo, that person who brakes hard, then accelerates to regain momentum and wastes energy in the process.

Cornering

It's one of our sport's most basic skills. Still, most of us could do it better. And corners come in all shapes and sizes—off-camber, decreasing radius, on lumpy pavement—which only amps up the challenge. But whatever type of turn you encounter, these essential tenets apply.

1. **MIND THE TERRAIN.** Look for and avoid sand, rocks, or cracks that could cause you to slip. After you know what the riding conditions are in a particular corner, you can slowly increase your speed each time.

2. **APPLY PRESSURE.** Do all your braking before the turn. Weight distribution is critical: To keep from sliding out, weight the front wheel by putting your hands in the drops of the handlebar with your

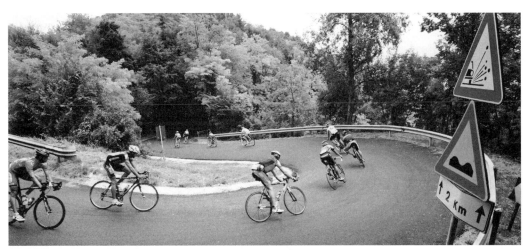

A road with switchbacks is a great opportunity to practice cornering.

elbows bent. Next, exert pressure with your outside hand and foot, creating angulation like you would in a ski turn. Don't try to pedal in a corner.

3. **LEAN THE MACHINE.** Release the brakes and start the turn by leaning the bike—not your body—into the turn. This can be accomplished by pushing lightly with your inside hand. Some call this *countersteering*. If the turn is tight or your speed increases, lean the bike farther in, and vice versa.

4. **AIM FOR THE INSIDE.** Carve a smooth arc through the apex of the turn: Start at the outside of the corner, near the center line. Aim toward the inside of the turn, then exit as far to the outside as possible. Do not cross the double yellow line.

5. **KEEP LOOKING . . .** in the direction you want to go. This will help you maintain a smooth line.

6. **MAKE YOUR EXIT.** As you come out of the turn, gradually straighten the bike until it's upright, then start to pedal again.

7. **MIND THE RAIN.** Painted lines, manhole covers, and oily pavement become slippery in wet conditions. Wet roads exaggerate everything you do: Braking while the bike is leaning will cause you to skid more easily, and sudden turning can make your wheels slip. So slow down.

DURING A GROUP RIDE OR EVENT

Alone or Leading a Group

The fastest way through a corner is whatever way you can go while still pedaling. Usually that's entering from the farthest outside edge, closing to the apex, then exiting to the farthest outside edge—essentially flattening the corner. When cornering on wide roads it's best to go from the outside to the inside or vice versa. This cuts down on the distance you travel. In a group, that can mean getting an extra pedal stroke or two of rest as the other guys catch up.

In a Pack

Follow the rider in front of you so you're still in his slipstream after the corner. If you don't trust him or you think you can go faster, take a line such as the outside-inside one. Remember: The smoother you are, the safer it is for everyone. Erratic braking is dangerous. Late in a race, I prefer to take an inside line. Most people exit to the outside, so it gets closed off. If you come outside-inside, there's always somewhere you can go. It's about courtesy. If you're not in the last few laps of a race, or nothing's on the line, there's no reason not to make room for someone. You're just making it dangerous if you don't.

Turns Sharper Than 90 Degrees

These are the types of corners you've got to nail, because they're more dangerous and they cost you more momentum, so you have to jump harder out of them. Exiting to the inside allows you to get back on the pedals faster. Being on the inside is paramount—the person on the outside gets squeezed out. When you're leading a pack, go outside-inside. In a pack, stay on the inside.

Being Forced to Change Lines

If someone forces you outside, you have to take a wider line. If someone passes you on the outside and comes in, you may have to tighten your line. You can scrub a little speed and tighten the turn, but I prefer to stand up so I can maneuver the bike beneath me and throw it back and to the inside of the corner, putting more of my weight over the front wheel. This is more about the handlebar than the body— you can rub shoulders or elbows, but you don't want to bump handlebars. You move the bike underneath you by shifting your weight, just for a moment, to give the person an exit lane.

Pro Tip

To make a wet corner less treacherous, make your turn as shallow as possible. Set up wide so you enter from a shallow angle, steer straight through the turn, then exit wide. In effect, this transforms one tight turn into two shallow ones.

Pedal Stroke

Pedaling in a simple circle is a complex thing, but mastering it can save energy, says biomechanist Todd Carver, director of fit for Retül, a professional bike fitting system. He says that with proper ankling (shown on page 104; not the injury-causing technique of the past), riders can churn out the same amount of power at a heart rate as many as 5 bpm lower. This stroke is for flat terrain at threshold, or time trial, intensity.

HIP-KNEE-ANKLE ALIGNMENT

Viewed from the front, your hip, knee, and ankle should line up throughout the pedal stroke. "You don't want knee wobble," says Carver. "Just think pistons, straight up and down." If you can't correct this, or if you experience knee pain when you try to restrict lateral movement, you may need orthotics or another type of biomechanical adjustment.

Zone 1

Known as the *power phase*, the portion of the pedal stroke from 12 o'clock to about 5 o'clock is the period of greatest muscle activity. "A lot of people think hamstrings are used only on the upstroke," says Carver, "but a good cyclist uses a lot of hamstring in the downstroke, because it extends the hip." The key to accessing the large muscles in the back of your leg is dropping your heel as you come over the top of the stroke, says Carver. "At 12 o'clock, your toes should be pointed down about 20 degrees, but as you come over the top, start dropping that heel so that it's parallel to the ground or even 10 degrees past parallel by the time you get to 3 o'clock." The biggest mistake Carver sees in novice riders: not dropping the heel enough in Zone 1.

Zone 2

Using the same muscles as in the power phase, but to a lesser degree, this phase acts as a transition to the backstroke. "As you enter Zone 2, think about firing the calf muscles to point your toe," Carver says. As you come through the bottom of the stroke, the toe should be pointed down 20 degrees. "This ankling technique transfers some of the energy developed in Zone 1 by the bigger muscles to the crank," Carver says. He uses the advice popularized by Greg LeMond: "Act like you're scraping mud off the bottom of your shoe."

Zone 3

Even though you feel like you're pulling your foot through the back of the stroke, you're not. "When you look at even the best cyclists, they're losing power on the upstroke," says Carver. "The pedal is actually pushing your leg up, so the goal is to lose as little power as possible and get that foot out of the way." One fun way to improve the efficiency of your upstroke is mountain biking. "The terrain keeps you honest," Carver says. "If you're focusing only on the downstroke, you'll lose traction and fall off your bike in steep sections." As for other exercises, Carver advises against single-leg pedal drills—"for recreation-level riders, they injure more people than they help"—but recommends hamstring- and glute-strengthening lifts as well as squats "done correctly, in a squat rack with someone showing you how."

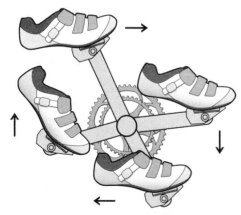

Clockwise from top: Zone 1, Zone 2, Zone 3, Zone 4

Pro Tip

The key to smooth, reliable, nondamaging gear changes when you're pushing hard is to ease your pedal pressure at the instant you move the shift lever. You need to lighten the load on the chain for about one revolution so it won't balk, crunch, or possibly break. Then hit the power again.

Zone 4

As you enter the second half of the upstroke phase, think about initiating your downstroke. "Many riders don't initiate early enough," says Carver, who often sees riders wait until 3 o'clock—but they should be starting before 12 o'clock. A tip: As you begin to come across the top of the stroke, think about pushing your knee forward, toward the bar. But only your knee, says Carver: "Your pelvis should remain a stable platform, not sinking down and not moving forward."

STILL PEDALING SQUARES? CHECK YOUR SADDLE POSITION. Proper bike fit, especially saddle height and fore-and-aft adjustment, is a prerequisite for a smooth pedal stroke. Without it, says Carver, you won't be even remotely as efficient as you could be. "If your saddle is too high, you're not going to be able to drive your heel effectively," he says. "If it's too low, you'll have knee pain." In the right position (knee over the ball of your foot with the pedal at 3 o'clock; knee slightly bent with the pedal at 6 o'clock), you'll maximize your energy output and also be able to adapt your ankling technique to different terrain, cadence, and effort levels.

Sprinting

In every group ride, there's always one yahoo who jumps first and wins the sprint for the town line sign or coffee stop. If that yahoo isn't you, you're missing out on the sweet music of your fellow riders muttering, cursing, wheezing, and panting as they struggle in vain to catch your wheel. There are no green sprinter's jerseys at stake, but who cares? You don't need no steenkin' jersey. Ah, but bragging rights—those are worth their weight in carbon fiber. (Don't aspire to out-muscle your friends? Say no more: The fine art of sprinting will also boost your total fitness and decrease your response time, which are benefits all riders will appreciate.) We asked Karen Bliss, a seventime US National Cycling Champion and one of America's best sprinters, about the secrets to explosive speed. She should know: During her 15-year career she won more criteriums and field sprints than any other female rider.

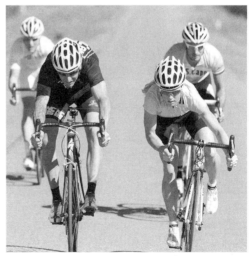

Not a natural sprinter? Be tactically smart.

Q: Are sprinters made or born?

KB: Sprinting is a learned discipline just like hill climbing or descending. Many cyclists convince themselves they can't sprint because they're not "built" for it—they lack the fast twitch muscle fibers, they lack the natural leg strength. But if you're not getting any faster, it's most likely you're not training properly. All cyclists, regardless of fitness level, can get faster and improve their overall cycling and fitness.

Q: How much is brawn, how much is brains?

KB: Even if you're not a natural sprinter, being confident and tactically smart can give you the edge over someone who's a better sprinter than you are. Body position is the first consideration. Get ready for the sprint by gripping the bar down in the curved section of your handlebar, where your fingers will be close enough to brake or shift gears when necessary. Your wrists should be straight, your elbows angled slightly outward, your shoulders square, and your head up.

Q: What's the anatomy of a sprint?

KB: There are two phases: Acceleration and top end. The acceleration or jump is the initial series of pedal strokes that get the bike up to speed. The top end is the highest speed, which should be timed to last through the finish line. The key is to pace yourself so you're still accelerating as you near the finish line—not topping out or slowing down. To jump, come up off the saddle and lean slightly forward. Apply full power to your dominant-side crankarm first while pulling up on the bar with your opposite hand. If your front wheel pops up or skitters, simply don't pull as hard. Keep increasing your leg speed with your elbows pointed out. Drop your head slightly. After the initial jump out of the saddle you can smoothly sit back down and continue to hold, or build speed for the duration of the distance.

Q: How do I pace my sprints?

KB: First you need to know how long you can hold your top speed. For professionals, most sprints begin somewhere around the 200-meter mark. When I raced, I would always study the end of a course beforehand to pick out a spot about 200 meters before the finish and etch that point into my mind. To find your pace, practice sprinting 50 meters, 100 meters, 150 meters, and 200 meters periodically to see how long you can hold your max speed. If you find your best sprint is 100 meters, then work that into your overall strategy.

Q: Will weight training make me faster?

KB: Sprinting requires very strong abdominal and back muscles, not so much for speed as for stability and precision. The abdominals and back muscles are "core" muscles that stabilize the upper and lower body while pedaling, as well as anchoring the body to the bike. Try sprinting with weak core muscle groups and your arms will feel like spaghetti looking for a plate. Follow a good abdominal and back routine 3 days a week.

Pro Tip

To develop a killer jump, practice standing starts. Here's how: Using a big gear such as the 53/19-tooth, roll to a slow speed, then accelerate at 100 percent effort as fast as possible for 20 to 30 pedal strokes. Begin with three to four sprints; build to six or seven. The first three pedal strokes are the most important. This is when the "sprint" message is transferred from brain to muscle fibers. The first stroke should be taken with your dominant leg, starting with the pedal at a 2 o'clock position.

Q: Why do I wobble when I sprint?

KB: A well-practiced sprinter makes that blur of speed look fluid and effortless—even while cranking the pedals in excess of 140 rpm. Less experienced riders will bounce up and down in the saddle when trying to turn the pedals at high speeds. One reason is they haven't developed the "muscle memory" that allows the pedal stroke to stay smooth and efficient rather than degenerate into a jerky push-pull, bobbing motion. Fortunately, you can train your muscles to fire and relax more quickly and efficiently. The trick is to spend some quality time every ride spinning at your fastest optimum leg speed—the point just before you usually begin to bounce in the saddle.

Descending

Going downhill is one of the hardest things for new cyclists to get used to. Why? The reason is simple: Speed scares people. There are even some pros who don't descend correctly, because they're either nervous or don't practice it enough. To start, familiarize yourself with the condition of the road surface by riding up the hill. Look for loose gravel on the shoulders, potholes or cracks on the pavement. Look also at the radius of the turns—do they follow a continuous arc, or do they become sharper during the middle of the turn? Are there sections that suddenly become steeper? As you gain experience, you

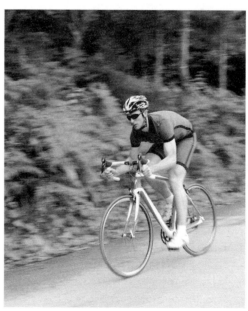

When heading down, keep your head up.

will be able to analyze on the fly, at speed. When you're ready to head down, follow these simple rules.

RIDE IN THE DROPS

With your hands on the lower part of the handlebar, your center of gravity is closer to the ground, like a race car. Also, your weight will be more evenly distributed between the front and rear wheels, which helps maintain traction, especially during braking and turning.

SCAN AHEAD

Look for danger signs so you have time to react. In turns, keep your eyes on the exit, which will help you carve a smooth, steady line all the way through.

STAY RELAXED

Start at the top of your body and let go of tension. Keep breathing, open your mouth to unclench your jaw, drop your shoulders, bend your elbows, release your death grip on the bar, uncurl your toes, and let your feet lie flat on the bottoms of your shoes.

USE SUBTLETY TO SLOW

Always anticipate what you'll need to do next. This will help you avoid sudden braking. For controlled slowing, gently squeeze both levers equally with 2- to 3-second pulses. Constantly riding the brakes on big descents can make rims overheat and possibly cause a blowout.

CORNER SMART

The biggest mistake people make descending is that they wait until they're in the middle of a turn to brake. Instead, scrub speed before the turn. If you have to brake in the turn, you didn't slow enough to begin with. Then push your outside pedal down (right turn, left foot down) with pressure on that foot. To initiate the turn, lean the bike—not your body—into the turn (right turn, lean bike right). The faster and sharper the turn, the more you'll lean the bike. This action is similar to downhill skiing: The lower body angulates into the turn while the upper body remains upright. To exit the turn, gently straighten the bike.

Pro Tip

On descents, your bike is much more stable when you're pedaling than when you're coasting.

Climbing

Climbing is funny: Some ascents are smooth and effortless, while others make you feel as if you're wresting an 800-pound walrus. The key, always, is rhythm. Here's how to find yours on any slope—from a gentle rise to Alpe d'Huez.

LONG, STEADY GRADES

On big climbs, effective climbing is about monitoring your effort so you never redline. Stay seated for prolonged periods. Slide back in the saddle a bit for leg extension and leverage. Relax your upper body and open your chest by pulling your shoulders back a bit. Hunching over inhibits breathing. Stand intermittently to give certain muscle groups (not to mention your butt) a break.

Your cadence should be high (not below 70 rpm; 80 to 90 is ideal). Mashing gears will fatigue you fast. Spinning—like a low-weight, high-rep weight workout—lets muscles recover faster. Amp up your effort for steeper pitches, then revert to a lower intensity.

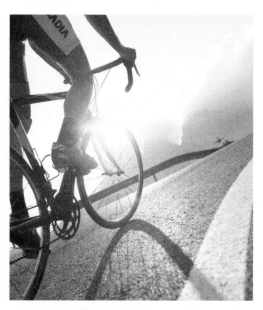

Hard climbs often lead to great views.

And keep your effort measured. Start by setting your pace roughly at what you think you can sustain, then back off a notch so you have some cushion if the grade steepens.

EXTRA CREDIT: Stretch on the bike. Stand and push hips forward to help your low back. To loosen your shoulders, slide backward and round your back. Pin your shoulders back to lengthen your neck.

ROLLERS

You'll go fastest on rolling terrain if you maintain your gearing and cadence as much as possible.

Stay in the gear in which you began climbing for as long as possible. Shift down only to keep your cadence steady. When you can see over the crest, shift up a gear to power over the top. Try to spin at 70 to 90 rpm. If you drop too low, you'll get bogged down; if you go too high, you'll unnecessarily lose momentum.

Attack the bottom of the roller at the same intensity as on the flats—but gradually increase the effort as you ascend. The ensuing descent lets you recover while maintaining speed.

Keep your hands on the hoods just as you would on the flats. Remain seated until your cadence drops by about 5 rpm, then stand; don't shift until your standing cadence drops another 5 rpm.

EXTRA CREDIT: Training? Use rollers as unstructured intervals. Pushing to the limit on one roller only to have to recover quickly for another will give you the ability to respond to attacks or put in your own double kick.

SHORT AND STEEP

Short inclines are best tackled aggressively. Start in the same gear as on the flats but be prepared to shift quickly and often to maintain cadence. You'll want to maintain a lower-than-normal cadence of 60 to 70 rpm. Spinning will cost you momentum on the steeps. You want to hammer the pedals and conquer these pitches as fast as possible. To do this, stand in the attack position, hands on hoods, body crouched. If seated, put your hands on the bar tops to open your chest and slide back slightly in the seat for maximum pedaling leverage.

Depending on the climb length, you'll either stand the whole time or alternate seated and standing. Stand when the gradient pitches up and sit when it backs off a notch, but keep the cadence consistent.

EXTRA CREDIT: When shifting, ease off the pedals a bit; the reduced tension will speed the shift and keep the chain in place.

CLIMB IN THE PACK

- **IF YOU'RE A WEAK CLIMBER,** start at the front and gradually drift back, so even as you lose ground you maintain contact with the group. This is more efficient than chasing from the back.

- **IF IT'S A COMPETITIVE RIDE,** don't get boxed in on the shoulder. And the shorter the hill, the harder you should work to keep an attacker's wheel. Or discourage attacks by setting the tempo.

- **IF YOU GET GAPPED,** keep your tempo steady. The pace up front might moderate, allowing you to catch back on.

- **WATCH OTHER RIDERS' FORM.** Jerky pedal strokes, hunched bodies, and other signs of deteriorating technique tell you they're tired.

Pro Tip

When climbing, visualize pedaling across the stroke rather than simply up and down. Strive to apply power horizontally through the bottom and top of the stroke.

FOR LONG-TERM GAINS

The obvious way to climb better is to climb more often. To improve your strength and stamina when the road turns up, add these drills to your hill days. For the best results, do them twice a week.

HILL ACCELERATIONS: Improve power on rolling hills, which last 1 to 2 minutes each but come at you one after another.

THE WORKOUT: Ride the majority of the roller at a steady and sustainable pace until you're 200 to 300 meters from the top. Stay seated and accelerate until you're about 10 seconds past the summit. Focus on increasing your cadence to create the initial acceleration, then use your gears to keep increasing speed as you reach and pass the top of the hill. Recover with 5 minutes of easy spinning and repeat. Novice riders should complete four hill accelerations, intermediate riders should complete two sets of four with 10 minutes of recovery between sets, and advanced riders can do two sets of six.

OVER UNDERS: These intervals alternate between a sustainable pace and a higher intensity to help you develop better power at your lactate threshold so you can handle changes on sustained climbs.

THE WORKOUT: During a 6-minute climb, ride "under" at a steady and sustainable climbing pace (86 to 90 percent of your maximum sustainable power output, or 92 to 94 percent of your maximum sustainable heart rate) for the first 2 minutes. For the "over" portion of the drill, accelerate to your maximum sustainable pace (95 to 100 percent of your maximum sustainable power output, or 95 to 97 percent of your maximum sustainable heart rate) for 1 minute. Return to your under intensity for another 2 minutes before accelerating again to your over intensity for the final minute. Stronger riders can add another cycle to make a 9-minute interval. Do three 6-minute intervals with 6 minutes of easy spinning recovery between them. If you do 9-minute intervals, keep recovery at 5 minutes.

HILL SPRINTS: These hard-charging intervals will give you the brute force you need to punch your way over short, steep walls. Just remember, after you hit the summit, use your gears to bring your cadence up so you don't get dropped after the climb.

THE WORKOUT: Find a short, steep hill with a flat road leading up to it. Ride toward the base of the hill at a moderate speed (15 to 20 mph). With your hands in the drops, get out of the saddle and start sprinting about 25 to 50 meters before you start going uphill. Continue sprinting for 10 seconds. Recover with 5 minutes of easy spinning between sprints. Novices should complete four hill sprints, intermediate riders should complete two sets of three sprints with 10 minutes between sets, and advanced riders should complete two sets of five sprints with 4 minutes between sprints and 8 minutes between sets.

Pro Tip

When climbing out of the saddle, if you feel your body bobbing too much, shift one gear harder. If you feel like you are excessively swinging your bike from side to side, shift one gear easier. These adjustments will give you an ideal balance of power and cadence.

Fast and Steady Win the Race

If you want to be first to the top of a climb or across the finish line, you have to train for it—these accomplishments aren't handed out to just anyone. Many riders don't do the intense training required to truly boost performance "because it hurts," says Jeb Stewart, owner of Endurofit Integrated Coaching Solutions in Tampa, Florida. If you want results badly enough, you'll endure the pain.

These four drills from Jeb Stewart and Andy Applegate, co-owner of VeloSports Performance Center in Asheville, North Carolina, will kick your butt while kicking your riding into a higher gear without giving you more than you can handle. Do two a week, choosing the ones that focus on your weakest areas. Bookend each workout with a 10- to 20-minute warm-up and cool down.

Improve Your: SPRINTING

"This workout touches on all aspects of sprinting, whether you need to accelerate quickly or make it to the line on a long 200- to 300-meter finish," says Stewart. "It will help make you faster, stronger, and able to lay down the power when it counts."

Warm up. Then do three 8- to 10-second jumps in the small chainring with 90 seconds between each to open up your legs and get

them ready to work. Then do these sprint sets: Three 8-second small chainring sprints at 130 to 150 rpm; three 15-second big chainring sprints at 120+ rpm; three 30-second big chainring sprints at 110+ rpm; three 10- to 15-second uphill sprints; three 15- to 30-second sprints. Allow at least 3 minutes recovery between repetitions and 5 minutes between sets. If you're just starting out, do just the first three sets and work up to five.

Improve Your: CLIMBING

Hilly races are brutal because you're always at or above threshold, says Applegate. These surges mimic racing pace efforts so you won't get shelled on race day.

For short-climb strength: Warm up, then head to a moderate hill (6 to 9 percent). Do seven 2-minute surges, building to a heart rate about 5 to 10 beats above your lactate threshold. If you are using power as a measurement, it's the average wattage you can sustain for 6 minutes. At 30, 60, and 90 seconds of each surge, attack out of the saddle for 10 pedal strokes. Recover for 4 minutes between surges. For long-climb strength: On a moderate climb (6 to 8 percent), do three 10-minute surges at lactate threshold heart rate or power. Every 2 minutes attack for 10 to 15 pedal strokes out of the saddle. After each, return to threshold heart rate/power (not below it). Recover for 10 minutes after each 10-minute effort.

Improve Your: **ATTACKING**

Success in cycling is all about your ability to redline and recover over and over again. "The following drill trains your body to tolerate the repeated anaerobic efforts of crits, fast group rides, and cyclocross racing," says Applegate.

Warm up, then ride as hard as humanly possible for 30 seconds. Recover for 30 seconds. Repeat 20 times, or for about 10 minutes. This one is best done with a friend or two so you have someone to push you to your limit on each effort.

Improve Your: **ENDURANCE**

Raise your lactate threshold and you'll raise your game. "These VO_2 max intervals deliver the biggest bang for your buck because they give you many of the training benefits of lactate threshold work but in less time, with less residual fatigue, and at a higher speed," says Stewart. "They help improve your lactate tolerance, time trialing speed, and breakaway riding ability."

Warm up, then do 3 to 5 minutes at lactate threshold followed by 5 minutes easy. Then do these maximum VO_2 efforts: Crank it up to maximum VO_2 heart rate (5 to 10 beats above lactate threshold heart rate, between time trial and all-out pace) and a 95 to 110 rpm cadence and hold for 3 to 6 minutes (depending on fitness). Recover 3 minutes.

Repeat two more times. That's one set. Do three sets with 5 minutes of recovery between sets.

Look Ma, No Hands!

Stay cool and hydrated and help—or impress—a friend with these on-the-roll maneuvers.

There are no time-outs on road rides. Everything you need to do—even things you don't—can be completed without stopping. Take the 1992 Tour de France, in which Frankie Andreu was descending the Col de la Croix de Fer with Motorola teammate Sean Yates. "I got on his wheel and we were flying, going white line to white line through switchbacks," recalls Andreu. "I'm just barely hanging on and all of a sudden Sean goes no-handed, reaches down and refastens his shoes." Here's how to take your mitts off the bar.

ONE HAND

Drinking and Eating

Keep your dominant hand on the handlebar. Pros: Keep your fingers on the brake hood, near the lever. Newbies, Keep yours on the bar tops, close to the stem, for greater control. Reach for your bottle or energy bar with your other hand. Holding the energy bar at the end, bite the seam corner and pull down to zipper open the wrapper. Biggest mistake is white-knuckling the bar, which can throw you off balance and exaggerates every minor bump.

Removing Knee Warmers

Keeping one hand on the handlebar, use the other to push one warmer down around your ankle, making a ring, like Mom used to before putting on your sock, says road and cyclocross pro Tim Johnson. Then clip your foot out, lift it, and pop the ring over your shoe. Ditto for the other warmer. Don't shift your weight, or you could lose your balance. "If I can't do it in one shot because of a corner or a pothole, I just leave it at my ankle until the timing is better," says Johnson.

The Helping Hand

To aid a bonked friend with a push, "use him or her to help you balance," says mountain bike veteran Hans Rey. For better leverage and a more stable position, move one hand to the center of your handlebar, just next to the stem. "Place your other hand, straight-armed, on the shoulder or low back, and push," says Rey.

Clearing Tire Debris

Reach down under your handlebar in front of your front brake and, using the web between your gloved thumb and index finger, gently brush the tire for several revolutions. For the rear tire, hook a thumb around the seatstay bridge so you don't accidentally pull your hand into the gap between the frame and rear tire. Duh: Don't ever do this without gloves.

NO HANDS

The Victory Salute

It may seem frivolous, but mastering this move helps build good one- and no-handed skills, says Johnson. "Plus, taking a win with one hand on the bar? Lame." To show off with style, work up a decent head of steam on an open road, then sit up and back with pedals horizontal. To keep your bike on course, clamp your knees around the top tube or keep pedaling (momentum helps you stay straight). Then stick 'em up.

Removing Arm Warmers

Use Johnson's "ring" technique, then sit up and pull the warmer off with your opposite hand.

Cornering

Practice on a straight, flat, or slightly downhill road: Start gently weaving from side to side, then gradually sit up and lighten your grip on the bar until only your fingertips are touching—you'll feel how you can subtly steer the bike just by shifting your hips. To steer right, put the left pedal down and rock your hips slightly to the left, and vice versa for the right.

Pacelining

The point of a paceline (when a group rides single file or two abreast) is to cover more

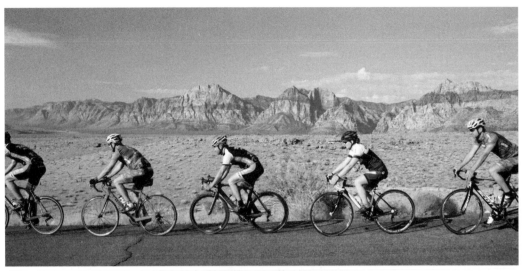

When in a paceline, always ride predictably.

ground with less effort. Each rider takes a turn at the front to block the wind, then rotates to the back and up through the line again. You conserve the most energy when you're riding about 6 inches behind the wheel in front of you—but that can feel scary at first.

MASTER IT: Practice with a small group, says Meredith Miller, who rides for Team TIBCO. This allows you to pull off and merge back in more often. Practice looking over the shoulder of the rider in front of you: Keep her back wheel in your peripheral vision instead of staring at it. Communication is key to having a good experience. Agree on a general (and steady) pace and make sure everyone knows not to speed up when they're in front.

STILL SHAKY? Do your arms and shoulders lock up and your wheel gets squirrelly any time a fellow rider comes within an arm's length? You may suffer from Pack-Riding Anxiety Disorder. This condition, also known as pelotonaphobia, often results in nervous looks from fellow cyclists during group rides and frequently causes ungainly gaps to open. Here's how to fix it: First of all, lay off the espresso. Then relax your arms, pedal smoothly, and focus on a spot over the shoulder of the rider in front of you (not on his rear tire). Once you're on his wheel, don't let your front wheel overlap it. Remember to breathe. Try not to brake (it affects everyone behind you), but if you must, do so gently—or just sit up a bit higher instead. Try riding with three friends in various formations at first.

Crash Course

When you start cycling, three things are bound to happen. First, you will try clipless pedals. Second, you will start receiving Nashbar catalogs. (Nobody knows why this is. It just happens.) Third, you will crash. Even though it's a virtual certainty, crashing is something for which we rarely prepare. And when I say "prepare," I don't mean "wear a helmet." No, to prevent crashing, you must expect it.

Here we present a primer on avoiding common scenarios and mistakes that can lead to falls. Remember these tips and practice a few key skills, and eventually they'll become hardwired for when you need them most. And for those moments when you go down, we offer a few tips on the fine art of limiting collateral damage.

MAKE THE SAVE

Six common causes of crashes—and some tips on how to avoid them.

Overlapped Wheels

HOW IT HAPPENS: Your front wheel passes the rear wheel of the rider in front of you, shrinking the amount of space and time you have to respond to whatever he does—and increasing the odds of bumping into him. "A guy at the front moves over 4 inches, and at the back it's 4 feet," says Tim Johnson, a pro who races for Cannondale/Cyclocrossworld.com. On Stage 9 of the 2011 Tour de France, three-time winner Alberto Contador overlapped wheels with Katusha's Vladimir Karpets. When Karpets inadvertently bumped him, Contador crashed and injured his knee—a mishap that may have contributed to his subpar finish.

AVOID IT: Watch the pack so that you know when riders up front are slowing. Overlaps often happen on corners, when riders scrub speed; anticipate this by coasting a bit into the corner. Leave enough room so that if the rider in front of you stands—which pushes his bike back underneath him about 6 inches—he won't overlap your front wheel.

TOO LATE? Feather the rear brake. Coast a pedal stroke or two. Don't swerve; the rider behind you is depending on your line. A bump won't necessarily knock you over. Practice absorbing contact in a park on your mountain bike, using flat pedals. Ride next to a friend and have him lightly bump you on your hip, says Roger Young, an Olympian who teaches track racing at the VELO Sports Center Velodrome in Los Angeles. Focus on holding your line with your hips, not your handlebar. If you try to correct your course using the bar, you'll veer off in the direction of the bump. Instead, correct at the hips and the bike will follow.

Keeping Your Head Down

HOW IT HAPPENS: During Stage 1 of the 2011 Tour de France, Astana's Maxim Iglinsky was riding at the edge of the pack on the shoulder. In a moment of inattention, he clipped a spectator, causing a domino-style crash that cost Contador and several other contenders more than a minute. "Sometimes we get too confident in the group," says Young. Riders also are prone to this when tired or distracted, leaving them vulnerable to the sudden appearance of pedestrians, parked cars, dogs, even garbage cans.

AVOID IT: Stay alert, always, even on familiar routes. Stop for caffeine if you need it. Fatigue can compromise pedaling, which profoundly affects your stability. Make sure your bike fits properly: You'll be less likely to ride with a slumped posture.

TOO LATE? Brake smoothly and stay in a straight line, especially on a group ride. Set your weight back a bit, which will help keep the bike upright and straight. If there's an obstacle ahead, try to lift your front wheel over it. If it's something like a garbage can, try to hit it with your hip first; it's closest to your center of gravity.

Hazardous Corners

HOW IT HAPPENS: Let us count the ways: An eddy of gravel or debris washed up in the bend. You're carrying too much speed. It's wet. You hit a slick painted line.

AVOID IT:

1. Be sensible and prioritize good form over sheer speed. If every corner is life-or-death, you'll be tense, which is counterproductive.

2. Keep your head up and look as far through the turn as you can. Avoid drifting through a left-hand turn and cutting across the turn lanes; you risk getting hit by oncoming traffic. Brake early, in the straightaway before the turn. Initiate the turn late and aim for a late apex. This keeps you from cutting across traffic and straightens out your exit.

3. Don't grab the brakes in a turn. You'll put extra force on the tires and push yourself to the outside of the turn.

4. If the roads are wet, let some air out of your tires. If you normally run them at 100 psi, go down to 90 psi to increase the amount of rubber on the road.

TOO LATE? Worst case, if you cut across a left-hand turn, you'll surprise someone coming at you in the turn lane. Stand the bike up to go straight—to the outside of the turn—then apologize to anyone behind you. If you have, say, gravel in your line and can't avoid it, just go through. "Stand the bike up slightly and point it straight," says Johnson. "Only change your line once you're through the debris."

Half-Wheeling

HOW IT HAPPENS: You're riding slightly ahead of the person next to you in a group or double paceline. The misaligned paceline, and the surges and ebbs in speed that result, can cause crashes behind you.

AVOID IT: Match gearing and cadence with the rider next to you. Stay away from hero pulls and other surges. It pisses off the people behind you, too.

TOO LATE? Soft-pedal a stroke or two to come even again. If the guy beside you surges, don't accelerate to meet him; he'll only creep ahead again each time you come even. Instead, hold the pack's pace and let him come back to you.

Riding Tense

HOW IT HAPPENS: If you're tight, every movement is magnified, says Young. You can't react quickly, and when you do, the reaction is exaggerated, which can send you into riders or obstacles around you.

AVOID IT: Proper bike fit? That's step one. Now go ride at a velodrome. With the fixed-gear, brake-free bike and pack of others, you'll develop spatial awareness and field vision and learn to scrub speed smoothly, stay locked on a wheel without fixating on it, and trade pulls. Most velodromes offer a basic track class with rentals. "Probably 85 percent of the people who ride here don't race track at all," says Young. "They just want to be better cyclists." No track nearby? Get a fixed-gear errand bike and try to use the drivetrain more than the hand brake. Bike polo also improves handling.

TOO LATE? Shake out your arms and roll your neck and shoulders. If you're riding on the brake hoods, hook your index and middle fingers over the front of the brakes—it's hard to put on a death grip with your pinkie. Change your hand position periodically.

Road Hazards

HOW IT HAPPENS: You or someone else hits a pothole or fishtails in gravel. Crashes in groups often look like ripples on a pond—one small move radiates outward, expanding, until someone's down.

AVOID IT: The safest spot to ride is almost always up front. In midpack, look ahead, beyond the rider in front of you. In turns, stay inside—physics takes crashes to the outside, so avoid the debris fan.

TOO LATE? Don't get caught gawking as the first rider goes down. Focus on an exit strategy—a way around or through the trouble ahead. What if riders are crashing around you? Point the bike straight, level the pedals, and flex your knees and elbows. You'll absorb impacts better and offer yourself a chance to ride out of the carnage.

LEGENDS OF THE FALL

It's all but impossible to push yourself technically without risking a crash, so don't worry about falling—worry about falling with grace. We asked these experts for advice: pro rider Tim Johnson, former pro Craig Lewis, and Shawn Crowder, a Hollywood-based film and television stuntman who specializes in falls and worked on the film *Avatar,* among others. The consensus: To get better at falling, fall under controlled conditions. Here's how.

DON'T FIGHT IT. "Often you can save a fall, but if you can't, just let it go," says Johnson. Particularly on the road, sometimes the safest approach is to simply lay down the bike—an approach that will seem less daunting if you've spent some time practicing falling. "If you fight the crash, you can end up causing more damage than was going to happen," Lewis says. That leads to point two.

USE PHYSICS. Sliding sucks because it means road rash. But it's better than a single hard hit because it disperses energy. "Never hit and stick," says Crowder. "The minute you hit the ground, keep rolling and moving; you never want to take 100 percent of the impact on one part of your body." In Lewis's experience, crashes happen in slow motion. "You can process a lot before you hit the ground," he says, "so you can do things like try to pick where you're going and aim for a soft landing spot."

HANG ON. Try to stay with your bike. Keep the bike at a relatively constant distance from your body to prevent hard and sharp parts flying at you.

BECOME DENSE. Johnson and Lewis extol the virtues of being loose, but not Crowder. "I actually believe in being tense," he says. However, there's a difference between being overly rigid and simply having your body prepared to take a hit. "If you get hit in the stomach, for example, you tighten up because the muscle deflects the impact. Basically, you want to be dense. If I'm doing a stunt like getting hit by a car, I'm a tight, taut ball."

PRACTICE. Take a gymnastics class. Yeah, that's right—just like you're 5 years old again. Many gyms nationwide offer adult classes that teach tumbling, rolling, and falling safely on mats. The Field House at Chelsea Piers in New York City (chelseapiers.com), for example, offers adult gymnastics classes starting at $28 per session. Or try skateboarding. No one falls more than skateboarders, and they frequently avoid injury, which speaks to one significant truth: The more you fall, the safer you'll fall. Plus, skateboarding relies on balance, which transfers to any sport. Camp Woodward (several locations, campwoodward.com) opens its skateboard camps to adults.

POSTCRASH CHECKLIST

Even if everything looks intact after a wreck, you might still be a catastrophe waiting to happen. A hairline crack can grow, a dent can buckle, a bend can break. Though it's hard to accept that your $100 helmet may be headed for the dump, remember that the only way to ride safely again is to do a thorough postcrash inspection. After you pick yourself up, complete this 10-minute inspection before your next ride.

HELMET. Assuming you're not wearing a multi-impact lid, one hit and your helmet is toast. Even if there is no visible damage to the shell, the foam layer's ability to protect your noggin from future hits has been compromised, but it may not be a total loss. Check with the manufacturer to see if it has a replacement policy.

FRAME. Clean it, then check for cracks, dents, and bulges. Examine around the head tube, chainstay, seatstay, brake bridge, bottom bracket, dropouts, and welds. If you notice anything amiss, have a professional assess it. *Warning*: Do not disregard a scratch in the paint. It could eventually result in rust or corrosion.

WHEELS AND BRAKES. Spin both wheels to make sure they are true and round. Wiggle them side to side to feel for play in the hubs. Check spokes to be sure that none has detensioned. Squeeze both brake levers to ensure that the pads are centered on and still contacting the rim.

STEERING AREA. Check that you didn't bend your handlebar. Then squeeze the front brake and rock the bike fore and aft to feel for play in the headset. On a mountain bike, check for looseness where the fork sliders enter the lowers. If anything is amiss, steering and balance will be out of line.

COMPONENTS. Check the rear derailleur and cranks; if they're bent, do not ride. Also check the saddle, seatpost, and pedals; if damaged, they must be replaced.

Just in Case

Yes, there is such a thing as cycling insurance. Bob Mionske, a former Olympic cyclist and the author of *Bicycling and the Law*, explains what you need to know—and why you might need it.

For years, I've advised bike riders to piece together cycling insurance through a combination of other types of policies, such as auto or homeowner's. Problem is, that can leave gaps in coverage, especially if you don't own a car. Comprehensive insurance policies for cyclists have never been available in this country—until now.

In 2011, I was contacted by a cyclist who also happened to be in the insurance business. He wanted to do something about the unmet need for bicycle insurance. We exchanged ideas, and he consulted members of the bike industry as well as national and regional cycling clubs and organizations. The result is Spoke Bicycle Insurance (spokeinsurance.com). Although originally it was available in only six states, it has since expanded nationwide.

DAMAGE FROM UNINSURED OR UNINSURED MOTORISTS. *This is the most important piece of insurance for any cyclist. It protects you* *in the event of a collision with an uninsured or hit-and-run driver. In the past, you needed to own an insured car in order to be covered. If you are a car-free cyclist, bike insurance is the only way to get this coverage.*

PERSONAL LIABILITY. *You'll be protected if you hurt someone while riding your bike, the same way an auto insurance policy covers you if you* *harm someone while driving a car. (Worth knowing: You may already be covered by your homeowner's or renter's insurance policy.)*

OTHER EXPENSES. *Bicycle insurance will cover your medical bills in the event of a crash, reimburse you for the value of your bike if it is stolen, and provide assistance if your bicycle breaks down during a ride.*

CHAPTER 8

Centuries

Some people are professional trainers and do little racing. But you can make the greatest gains through competition. I never would have realized my potential if it weren't for racing. There's nothing like it to push you. It improves fitness and bike handling. You find yourself at speeds you would never attain in training.

—NED OVEREND, US PROFESSIONAL CROSS-COUNTRY MOUNTAIN BIKE RACER, FORMER WORLD CHAMPION, AND MULTI-TIME NATIONAL CHAMPION

RIDING 100 MILES IN A SINGLE DAY IS A RITE OF PASSAGE FOR many cyclists. Although it may seem unimaginable, as long as you have a solid game plan, you'll be able to attain your goal—whether you're supporting a cause, enjoying a fun day with friends, trying to achieve a personal best, or all of the above. Below is a handbook for completing your first century, from pre-race prep to what to eat on the big day—even some last-minute advice for people who may have, um, procrastinated a bit on training.

Make Every Mile Count

Finishing a century means making the best choices before and during each of those 100 miles. With planning and attention to detail, you'll minimize mistakes and arrive at the finish line well before the food tent (or your body) is broken down.

PREP BIKE AND BODY

About a week before your event, take your bike to a trusted mechanic for a tune-up. If you're doing your own maintenance, be sure to address these key things: Confirm that the bike is shifting and braking smoothly and that the bolts securing the stem and headset are tight. Also pay attention to the places where the bike meets your body or the road: saddle, pedals and cleats, bar, and tires. Check for loose bolts, worn rubber, and peeling tape and make whatever repairs are necessary. On your training rides, practice skills such as cornering, braking, riding in a group, and eating and drinking on the bike.

PLAN AHEAD

Check the ride's web site for information on aid station locations, foods offered, the course profile, elevation, difficult segments, predicted weather conditions, parking, and instructions for nonriding spectators. Do this well in advance of event morning. Not only will it make for a less stressful ride, but it will also allow you to simulate event day

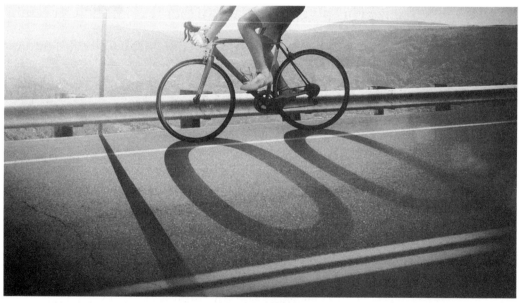

Triple-digit ride? NBD.

(including what and when you'll eat) in training. Also, don't introduce new gear or foods on race day. I can't tell you how many times I've seen otherwise well-prepared individuals sabotage their day by using an unfamiliar energy drink that upset their stomach or a new pair of shoes or saddle that caused pain 20 miles into the ride.

SPACE OUT FUEL

Stuffing yourself full of calories before the ride will divert blood to your stomach, which weakens your legs and slows you down. Instead, eat a carbohydrate-rich breakfast of 400 to 500 calories 2 to 3 hours before the event. Then aim to eat and drink 200 to 300 calories every hour thereafter.

KEEP A STEADY FLOW

Consume at least one 24-ounce bottle of energy drink per hour (more if it's hot) to provide electrolytes and a few carbohydrates. Choose a flavor that will entice you to sip often.

PEDAL YOUR PACE

The biggest newbie mistake is letting yourself be seduced into speeding along with faster riders early in the day, only to crack 60 miles in. Fall in with riders who pedal your pace and avoid going into the red (feeling breathless) for the first 50 miles. You'll finish fresh and strong.

MOVE AROUND

Avoid aches and pains in your neck and back by changing your hand position often and standing out of the saddle to stretch periodically.

KEEP IT SHORT

Take advantage of rest stops to use the bathroom, refill bottles, stretch, and grab some food. But don't linger. A stop that lasts more than 10 to 15 minutes will cause your legs to stiffen up and make it harder to get going again.

SKIP THE EARLY REST STOP

You shouldn't need to refill bottles for at least 20 miles, and you won't need to stop for calories in the first 30 to 40 miles of the ride. Skipping the first stop can save time and give you a jump on a lot of other riders, which means better food choices and smaller crowds when you pull into the later stops.

Pro Tip

WEAR OUT YOUR SHIFTERS. You have lots of gears for a reason: to keep your cadence in the sweet spot. For silky-smooth gear changes, remember to shift before a punchy climb, sprint, or tight switchback.

How to Eat for 100

A few hours on the bike will suck your glycogen stores dry; even a leisurely century burns about 4,000 calories. To fuel your 100-mile effort, follow this eating guide from Monique Ryan, RD, author of *Sports Nutrition for Endurance Athletes.*

2 DAYS BEFORE

Start loading carbs. That doesn't mean letting loose at Louie's Bakery. Eat meals that are

CRASH-COURSE CENTURY TRAINING

YOUR PLAN WAS TO BE TRIPLE-DIGIT FIT by September. Now that 100-miler you registered for light-years ago is a calendar flip away, and you've barely cracked 40. Do this century crash course (only if your fitness base includes a few rides a week), and you'll be ready to roll.

SHOOT FOR 65

COACHES ADVISE THAT YOU SHOULD BE ABLE to do a 75-mile ride before your century. But you can squeak by with 65 if you take it easy; you can increase your weekly long ride by a safe 10 to 15 percent for 4 weeks. Your schedule: Week 1, 45 miles; week 2, 51 miles; week 3, 57 miles; week 4, 65 miles.

ONE STEADY, ONE SPEED, ONE SPIN

RIDE 3 TO 4 DAYS A WEEK between now and the event: ride long one day, at a fast pace another, with one or two easy-spin days in between. Speed work improves endurance because your body learns to recover faster, and it helps you tackle headwinds and hills. Try this: Warm up for 20 minutes, ride fast for 20, cool down for 20. Inch up the mileage on your midweek rides by a mile or two as you progress toward the event.

TAKE YOUR TAPER

DON'T CRAM IN MILES THE WEEK BEFORE the ride. Keep your rides short so your body can be rested and ready.

KEEP IT CASUAL

AVOID INJURIES BY STARTING OUT SLOWLY AND spinning for the first 50 to 60 miles. Use the rest stops often to stretch and fuel; limit pit stops to 10 minutes.

carb heavy, such as pastas, whole grain cereals, couscous, brown rice, and whole grain bread, as well as beans, bananas, and sweet potatoes.

THE NIGHT BEFORE

Eat an easily digested meal that you've had a million times, such as spaghetti. Now is not the time to experiment with new sauces or anything that might upset your system. "And stay away from really high-fiber foods that will sit in your stomach and cause distress on the ride," Ryan says. "Be done with your meal by 9 p.m."

THE MORNING OF YOUR RIDE

No matter what you ate last night, your glycogen stores will be half empty when you wake up. "Your morning meal keeps you from feeling hungry," Ryan says. Two hours before start, have some oatmeal—it's easy to digest yet gives even, lasting energy. Aim for a bowlful with a banana along with some juice and coffee.

REST STOP #1 AT 20 MILES

You shouldn't be too depleted yet. This is a good time for 30 to 60 grams of easily digested carbohydrates: a sports drink and half an energy bar. Also, always pack a few snacks, no matter how well-supported the ride.

REST STOP #2: LUNCH AT 45 MILES

You've been on the road about 3 hours and your muscle glycogen stores are depleted. Have a peanut butter and jelly sandwich with some juice, fig bars, and potato chips. "Emphasize carbohydrates and protein," Ryan says. Other smart choices include turkey subs, hummus wraps, and bagel sandwiches.

REST STOP #3 AT 65 MILES

This is no-man's-land. You're not close enough to the end to get juiced, but you're too far in to be fresh. Many cyclists get psychologically tired in the 60-something stretch. The solution: chocolate! "Eat a Milky Way," Ryan says. "Buy one on the way or freeze it the night before if the weather's not too hot."

REST STOP #4 AT 85 MILES

Hydration is your priority. "You're in the heat of the day, and your sweat losses are probably catching up with you," Ryan says. "Pack a little of your favorite powdered energy drink in a Ziploc bag and mix it up at this stop. It'll replenish you for the final miles."

THE FINISH AT 100 MILES

Stretch out. Within 20 minutes of finishing, find a nice restaurant and eat a high-carb, moderate-protein meal, such as chicken with linguini, to restock your glycogen stores while your muscles are at their hungriest.

Seeing Double

If you've ridden a century or two—and liked it—you're probably ready to tackle a double century. The event itself may be the easy part: Doing a double requires meticulous preparation and logging lots of extra training miles. Here's your guide.

DO YOUR HOMEWORK

Study the route, ride reports, and support information from the organizer. Use your training rides to test your drinks and food, along with the clothing you plan to wear, to find out what works. "Riders come in with miles in their legs but aren't prepared to deal with cramps, hot spots, and problems with drinking," says Jim Cummins, executive director of the Dirty Kanza, a 200-mile ride through the remote Flint Hills of Kansas.

GET COMFORTABLE

Take care of nagging pains before the event. You may need to adjust your saddle, handlebar, and cleat positions. Any discomfort you feel on these contact points at mile 80 will be magnified by mile 120. Switch to durable tires to minimize your risk of flatting, and if your event is hilly, consider a compact, triple, or even a 34/27 setup to help you spin with less effort.

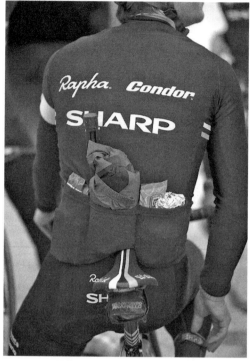

Being prepared is half the battle.

DEVISE A CARRYING STRATEGY

Figure out what to stow where in your jersey pockets. Anything you'll want while rolling, such as food or a camera, should go in the pocket you are most comfortable accessing with one hand. You might also want to try different ways to carry additional fluids, such as a frame bag or hydration pack.

VARY YOUR TRAINING

Include hills, tempo efforts, and sprints, along with slow, long, and short rides. And remember to rest for a day or two every week.

FINISH STRONG

These event-day strategies will keep you happy in the saddle and able to finish all 200 miles feeling like you could tackle more.

- Start slow and maintain a consistent pace.
- Ride in a paceline to conserve energy.
- Limit breaks to no more than 10 minutes so your muscles don't feel tight when you remount.
- Stand up out of the saddle from time to time.
- Plan to eat about 300 calories an hour, including plenty of easy-to-digest carbohydrates in the form of sports drinks, bars, and gels.

ESSENTIAL GEAR FOR THE LONG HAUL

You don't have to carry all of this gear in your jersey pockets, but bring them to the race just in case.

- Lights and spare batteries
- Arm and leg warmers, cap, gloves, and vest
- A chain breaker, tire levers, pump or CO_2, and a hex wrench sized for every bolt on your bike
- Two to three spare tubes
- Money, ID, insurance info, sunscreen, and phone

Training Plans

FINISH YOUR FIRST CENTURY

A 100-mile ride may seem like it requires hundreds of training hours, but the good news is that short, intense efforts trump volume: You don't need to ride far every day, and even if you plan to take it easy during the event, don't pedal only at that pace during training. You will improve your overall cruising speed more effectively by doing three rides of 60 to 90 minutes each week that include high-intensity intervals than by going long only on the weekends. This plan is for cyclists who currently average 40 to 50 miles per week or who are by nature more tentative.

Workouts

EASY: A leisurely ride. If you need to adjust the schedule due to time crunches or other commitments, always make sure the easy day follows a high-mileage or brisk day.

PACE: The average speed you're aiming for on century day.

BRISK: Two to three mph faster than your average century speed.

After finishing your first century, complete your second one faster with our advanced training plan at Bicycling.com/centuryplan.

Your Century Training Plan

WEEK	MONDAY	TUESDAY	WEDNESDAY	THURSDAY	FRIDAY	SATURDAY	SUNDAY
1	**Easy** 6 miles	**Pace** 10 miles	**Brisk** 12 miles	Rest day	**Pace** 10 miles	**Pace** 30 miles	**Pace** 9 miles
Weekly total: 77 miles							
2	**Easy** 7 miles	**Pace** 11 miles	**Brisk** 13 miles	Rest day	**Pace** 11 miles	**Pace** 34 miles	**Pace** 10 miles
Weekly total: 86 miles							
3	**Easy** 8 miles	**Pace** 13 miles	**Brisk** 15 miles	Rest day	**Pace** 13 miles	**Pace** 38 miles	**Pace** 11 miles
Weekly total: 98 miles							
4	**Easy** 8 miles	**Pace** 14 miles	**Brisk** 17 miles	Rest day	**Pace** 14 miles	**Pace** 42 miles	**Pace** 13 miles
Weekly total: 108 miles							
5	**Easy** 9 miles	**Pace** 15 miles	**Brisk** 19 miles	Rest day	**Pace** 15 miles	**Pace** 47 miles	**Pace** 14 miles
Weekly total: 119 miles							
6	**Easy** 11 miles	**Pace** 15 miles	**Brisk** 21 miles	Rest day	**Pace** 15 miles	**Pace** 53 miles	**Pace** 63 miles
Weekly total: 178 miles							
7	**Easy** 12 miles	**Pace** 15 miles	**Brisk** 24 miles	Rest day	**Pace** 15 miles	**Pace** 59 miles	**Pace** 18 miles
Weekly total: 143 miles							
8	**Easy** 13 miles	**Pace** 15 miles	**Brisk** 25 miles	Rest day	**Pace** 15 miles	**Pace** 65 miles	**Pace** 20 miles
Weekly total: 153 miles							
9	**Easy** 15 miles	**Pace** 15 miles	**Brisk** 25 miles	Rest day	**Pace** 15 miles	**Pace** 65 miles	**Pace** 20 miles
Weekly total: 155 miles							
10	**Easy** 15 miles	**Pace** 15 miles	**Brisk** 25 miles	Rest day	**Pace** 10 miles	**Easy** 5 miles	Race day
						Note: If your event is on a Saturday (most are on Sunday) simply shift the last week's schedule back a day. (Take Wednesday off and ride 10 miles on Thursday and 5 on Friday.)	
Weekly total: 170 miles							

CHAPTER 9

Charity Rides and Gran Fondos

Racing, on any level, seeks a balance within us. For every moment of hassle and pain, there is one of revelation and joy. For my money, I'll take the bad road food with the good sunsets, the injured weak days with the winning sprints, and the long hot drives with the two hours of playing in the dirt. Is it worth it? Always.

—MIKE FERRENTINO, CYCLING WRITER

AMERICAN CYCLISTS WHO WANT TO RIDE IN AN ORGANIZED event typically have two choices: They can plunk down $70 for a USA Cycling license and take their chances in the competitive mayhem of a race, or they can raise $100 or more for a charity and join the legions of tourists on an untimed Sunday ride.

What if your riding sensibility lies somewhere between the two? What if you're not fit enough to race competitively but like the *idea* of racing: riding in a paceline on a challenging course, for a distance that feels a little too far to be going that fast, with solid support and controlled traffic. Enter the gran fondo, or "big ride," a type of timed, mass-cycling event that takes recreational pedaling to a new level.

Whether you're looking for a fun way to give back or a simulated race, this chapter will prepare you for the varied distances of both challenges.

Charity Rides

Want to use your passion for a purpose? Hop onto the charity ride bandwagon this year. Charity rides draw big crowds by welcoming everyone from families out for a few miles to best friends pushing it for 7 straight days in honor of someone or something they believe in. And that's the idea: Through entry fees and fund-raising, these events benefit cancer research, children's hospitals, humane societies, and more.

Unlike a race, for which solid fitness and pack-riding skills are a must, bike rides for a cause are pleasantly noncompetitive. Rides vary in days and distance, and for many signing up is great motivation simply to enjoy time on the bike, both during the event and on conditioning rides leading up to it. Choose an

event that allows you sufficient time to raise the necessary funds. Once you make your choice, sign up before hesitation sets in. Worst case: If you bail, your registration fee will still go toward the cause.

Nervous about making the commitment? Plan to ride with at least one other person. Friends mean training partners, race-day camaraderie and support, and collective fund-raising efforts (a raffle, yard sale, or potluck with a monetary donation). "Riding with a friend helps you overcome fears," said Richard Fries, director of rides marketing for the Best Buddies Challenge. "New riders might worry about getting a flat or how they look in spandex." A buddy can provide moral support or be a sounding board for concerns.

For ride tips, fund-raising advice, and multi-distance training plans, read on.

PICK YOUR PASSION: WHICH RIDE SHOULD YOU DO?

Cyclists take many things into account when choosing a ride to support: personal connection to the cause, location, the size of the post-ride burrito. Also consider how the beneficiary spends your money. Charity Navigator (charitynavigator.org) evaluates more than 5,300 organizations and doesn't charge for access to its listings.

Charity Navigator rates nonprofit organizations based in the United States that receive more than $500,000 in public support each year on a scale of zero to four stars. (About 1,700 groups currently merit the highest rating.) It does not rate hospitals, private or community foundations, colleges or universities, PBS stations, land trusts or preserves, and religious organizations (such as the Salvation Army) that are exempt from filing IRS Form 990, which Charity Navigator uses to determine ratings.

Even if your cause of choice isn't listed, you can ask questions to determine a nonprofit's worthiness. (Federal law requires that charities make 3 years of financial data publicly available.) Here are some factors Charity Navigator takes into account.

Organizational Efficiency

What percentage of expenses are relate to programs, as opposed to administration and fund-raising? Ideally, it's 75 percent or more.

Fund-Raising Efficiency

How many cents does the organization spend to raise each dollar? Fewer than 10 is commendable.

Growth

Are revenues—and services—increasing over time?

Working Capital

How long could the charity sustain its programs without raising more money? The answer should be at least a year.

Pro Tip

When you start to feel stressed and overwhelmed by a hard pace, try this breathing technique: Instead of actively drawing air into the lungs then, passively letting it out (our normal pattern), push the air out and let it naturally flow back in. Bonus: Because of how you activate your lungs to do this, it also helps you get into a low riding position and maintain a flatter back.

ACE YOUR FUND-RAISING GOAL

Charity rides are a popular way to test yourself and help out a cause, but it's not always easy to ask people to donate. Shannon Gilmartin of Orchard Park, New York, knows a thing or two about drumming up support; she has raised more than $30,000 for the Dempsey Challenge, a charity ride in Maine that supports the Patrick Dempsey Center for Cancer Hope and Healing. Here are a few of her secrets.

Sell Stuff

People are more likely to donate if they get something in return. "I like to bake," Gilmartin says. "So I organize a Confections for Cancer Patients campaign. All proceeds from my cakes, cookies, and pies go to the Dempsey Challenge."

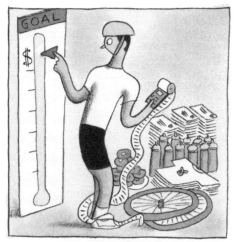
Get creative with your fundraising efforts to achieve your goal easily.

Organize a Raffle

"I had one of my most effective fund-raisers after I bought scrubs and paired them with a *Grey's Anatomy* script I won in a Twitter contest," Gilmartin says. "I took them to one of Patrick Dempsey's car races and waited in the autograph line. Then I raffled off the signed memorabilia and raised over $2,000."

Be Crazy

The wackier you can be, the more attention you will bring to your cause. "One year I organized a Pie Me in the Face game," Gilmartin says. "People donated money for a chance to throw a whipped cream pie at me." Share the pictures on social media sites to raise awareness and engage potential supporters.

25- TO 50-MILER TRAINING PLAN

Middle-distance charity rides are a great way for beginner cyclists to get their feet wet in endurance cycling. If your chosen nonprofit doesn't provide a training plan for the event, these workouts will get you fit in under 10 hours a week.

GROUP RIDE RULES

IF YOU DON'T HAVE A LOT OF experience riding in a pack, follow these guidelines.

BE PREDICTABLE: Hold your line and use signals. Avoid sudden braking, swerving, or accelerating in a paceline.

LOOK AHEAD: Don't just stare at the wheel in front of you. Train your eyes beyond the rider and watch for terrain changes.

KEEP THE PACE: Stay even with your fellow riders. Too tired to work? It's okay to sit in at the back.

Workouts

Active Recovery Pace

Rate of perceived exertion: 1 to 4

A very slow pace; you're able to hold a conversation

Endurance Pace

Rate of perceived exertion: 5 to 6

A pace that you can endure and speak; typical Saturday-ride effort

Overall Endurance Pace+

Endurance pace with 4 × 6-minute intervals at a rate of perceived exertion of 9 (a pace at which you can't speak, but not quite all out).

Pro Tip

STICK WITH YOUR GROUP. Whether you're embarking on a 500-mile charity ride or racing Paris–Nice, there's safety in numbers. Teammates and friends can pull if you're feeling tired, share their food, or help fix a mechanical problem. "I've seen this so many times," says Chris Horner, a 2013 Vuelta a España winner. "A guy is leading the race and is really strong and so he goes into a breakaway. But what happens if he crashes or flats? He is all alone. Stay with your group as long as possible." Be sure to shift your weight behind your saddle to prevent yourself from sailing over the handlebar.

Your 25- to 50-Miler Training Plan

WEEK	MONDAY	TUESDAY	WEDNESDAY	THURSDAY	FRIDAY	SATURDAY	SUNDAY
1	Rest day	**Endurance** 1 hr	**Endurance** 1 hr	**Active recovery** 1 hr	Rest day	**Endurance** 2 hr	**Active recovery** 1 hr
2	Rest day	**Endurance** 1.5 hr	**Active recovery** 1 hr	**Endurance** 1 hr	Rest day	**Endurance** 2.5 hr	**Endurance** 1 hr
3	Rest day	**Endurance** 1.5 hr	**Active recovery** 1 hr	**Endurance** 1.5 hr	Rest day	**Endurance** 3 hr	**Endurance** 1.5 hr
4	Rest day	**Endurance** 1.5 hr	**Active recovery** 1 hr	**Endurance** 1.5 hr	Rest day	**Endurance** 3 hr	**Active recovery** 1 hr
5	Rest day	**Overall Endurance Pace+** 1.5 hr	**Active recovery** 1 hr	**Active recovery** 1 hr	Rest day	**Event**	

MULTIDAY RIDE TRAINING PLAN

Looking forward to that tour, but not really sure how to get ready for it? Here's a plan that can help you get ready for those day-after-day miles. *Note:* This is an ambitious plan that was designed for someone who rides regularly—a couple group rides per week and a long ride of 2 or more hours on weekends. So pay attention to how you feel. If you get overtired, feel drained, or just grow sick of the bike, take an extra rest day to recover a bit more.

Workouts

EASY: This is essentially a recovery ride. No hard efforts. Keep your cadence high.

BASE: This is minimal-effort riding. Judge by your breathing: It should be steady but relaxed, and you should be able to carry on a conversation.

TEMPO: This is a level above base. Breathing is quicker and the pace is harder. On a scale of 1 to 10, this effort would rate about a 7.

THRESHOLD: Just less than all-out. Breathing is quick, and your legs are likely burning. On a scale of 1 to 10, this effort would be an 8 or 9.

Multiday Ride Training Program

WEEK	MONDAY	TUESDAY	
1	Rest day	**Base** with 3 × 15 min Tempo 1 hr, 15 min	
2	Rest day	**Base** with 3 × 15 min Tempo 1 hr, 15 min	
3 Max time/ effort week	Rest day	**Base** with 4 × 15 min Tempo 1 hr, 30 min	
4 Recovery week	Rest day	**Base** 1 hr	
5	Rest day	**Base** with 2 × 25 min Tempo 1 hr, 30 min	
6 Max time/ effort week	Rest day	**Base** with 3 × 20 min Tempo 1 hr, 30 min	
7	Rest day	**Base** with 2 × 30 min Tempo 1 hr, 30 min	
8 Recovery week before event	Rest day	**Base** with 2 × 10 min Tempo 1 hr	

	WEDNESDAY	THURSDAY	FRIDAY	SATURDAY	SUNDAY
	Base 1 hr	**Base** with two 3 × 15 min Tempo 1 hr, 15 min	**Base** 45 min	**Base** with 20 min Tempo and 3 × 10 min Threshold 2 hr	**Base** 3 hr
	Base 1 hr	**Base** with two 20-min efforts (15 min Tempo, 5 min Threshold. Repeat.) 1 hr, 30 min	Easy ride or rest day	**Base** with 30 min Tempo and 3 × 15 min Threshold 2 hr, 30 min	**Base** 3 hr
	Base 1 hr	**Base** with two 30-min efforts (20 min Tempo, 10 min Threshold. Repeat.) 1 hr, 30 min	**Base** 1 hr	**Base** with 30 min Tempo and 3 × 15 min Threshold 2 hr, 30 min	**Base** 3 hr, 30 min
	Easy 30 min	**Base** 1 hr	Rest day	**Base** 1 hr, 30 min	**Base** 2 hr
	Base 1 hr	**Base** with two 25-min efforts (15 min Tempo, 10 min Threshold. Repeat.) 1 hr, 30 min	Easy ride or rest day	**Base** with 30 min Tempo and 3 × 15 min Threshold 2 hr, 30 min	**Base** 3 hr, 30 min
	Base 1 hr, 15 min	**Base** with two 30-min efforts (20 min Tempo, 10 min Threshold. Repeat.) 1 hr, 30 min	**Base** 1 hr	**Base** with 40 min Tempo and 3 × 15 min Threshold 2 hr, 30 min	**Base** 4 hr
	Base 1 hr	**Base** with two 30-min efforts (20 min Tempo, 10 min Threshold. Repeat.) 1 hr, 30 min	**Base** 1 hr	**Base** with 40 min Tempo and 3 × 15 min Threshold 2 hr	**Base** 4 hr
	Rest day	**Base** with 2 × 5 min Tempo, 2 × 5 min Threshold. 1 hr	Rest day	**Base** with 2 × 3 min Tempo and 2 × 3 min Threshold 1 hr	Event start

continued on next page . . .

Gran Fondos

Often called *cyclosportives*, these events are popular in Italy, France, and the United Kingdom. The rides typically follow the classic courses used in Grand Tours and other races, allowing everyday riders to pretend to be pro for a day. The concept isn't entirely new here in the United States: The Univest Grand Prix Cyclosportif, first held in Souderton, Pennsylvania, in 1998, claims to be the first such event on American soil. Now it's starting to catch on.

Gran fondos usually offer a choice of routes. They're normally at least 100 miles long, with plenty of difficult climbs. The *medio*, or medium, course averages about 62 miles. There's also often a flatter, shorter route for beginners. Unlike most century rides, gran fondos are usually timed. The top riders are there to win—former pros sometimes even make a living by riding gran fondos as part of a sponsored team, and some events award medals to anyone who finishes within certain time limits. Competition is less of a factor in the United States, where most courses can't be completely closed to cars. However, many American gran fondos will include a time-trial section, such as a timed climb.

While American gran fondos may not be able to provide the same race atmosphere as their foreign counterparts, their organizers have been careful to import the fondo's most appealing attributes: well-stocked aid stations, sumptuous postevent meals, and a chance to share the road with the likes of Levi Leipheimer or George Hincapie.

Sound good? Here's what you need to know to complete your first fondo or ride your next one faster.

A Century vs. a Fondo

While the typical gran fondo will set your bank account back a bit more than the average 100-miler, the Italian import may soon outpace the century in popularity. Which one's right for you? Compare them below.

RACE	AVERAGE COST	SCHWAG	VIBE	POSTRACE CHOW
Century	$44	Socks, maybe a T-shirt	Mellow club ride that lasts all day	Most offer pizza, pasta, and subs plus an energy drink to wash it down
Gran fondo	$101	Socks—plus a finisher's medal, commemorative jersey, and age-group awards	Similar to a race, complete with a mass start, timing chips, screaming fans, and cowbells	A foodie's fantasy: artisanal breads and cheeses, gourmet pizza, local wines, handcrafted beers

GET YOUR GEAR FONDO READY

What works on your Thursday-night club ride might not be good for 7-plus hours in the saddle with 6,000 feet of elevation gain. Try these tips.

Get a Bike Fit

You want a setup that keeps you comfortable and supple on the bike but aggressive enough to push when you need to, says Marc Bavineau, a former national cyclocross champion and former USA Cycling mechanic in Europe. Even if you're comfortable on the bike you ride regularly, take it to a fit expert (either a coach or certified fitter at your local bike shop) to make course-specific tweaks.

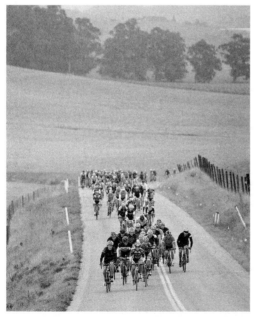

Gran frondo literally means "big ride."

DID YOU KNOW . . .

THE TERM *GRAN FONDO* COMES FROM CROSS-COUNTRY skiing events longer than 40 kilometers. Cycling adopted the name in the 1980s when long-distance, performance-oriented amateur group rides became popular in Italy and elsewhere in Europe.

Go Low

Grades sharper than 15 percent are not uncommon in fondos. Choose a gear you can spin, not mash, since anything in the steep zone puts you at risk for exploding. Marti Shea, a repeat winner at New Hampshire's Mt. Washington Hillclimb, advises a lower gear ratio. "It allows inexperienced climbers to find the gear they feel comfortable in," Shea says.

Make Your Feet Happy

After long hours in the saddle, riders sometimes notice soreness in the ball of the foot, where the cleat attaches to the shoe. Look out for this in training. Consider tweaking your cleat position back a tad to let you turn the pedals more comfortably on long, steady grades, says Bavineau. You may need to try different cleats, pedals, or shoes—or all three.

ACHIEVE YOUR BEST FINISH

Get the results you want with these simple strategies.

Make a Game Plan

After you choose your fondo, download the course map and study both the hill profiles and the route. Try to train on similar terrain. Riders who crack during a fondo haven't practiced on climbs like the ones they'll find on the course, which can exceed a 10 percent grade. The first hour of the race is the toughest. It's furiously fast, and a two-lane road will be jammed tight, 20 riders across. It's crazy, but you'll survive if you don't stress about the chaos.

Know How You're Being Scored

Organizers base results on timed climbs, a single time for the entire course, or both. They'll generally post multiple rankings, including listings by age and gender. Find out ahead of time to plan your strategy.

Wear Second Skins

Fondo conditions vary mightily, from broiling heat to icy fog. You won't stay at elevation long, so pack arm warmers and a simple vest or jacket. If the course has long descents, stay warm by putting on your jacket and vest at the top of the climb. It's a minute well spent. Also, stay as cool as you can while riding uphill. Open your jersey and roll down your arm warmers. Remove your jacket even if it's drizzling. Heating up on climbs will only slow you down. Guys, you'll also want well-broken-in bibs with a deep cut at the waist to allow easy pit stops.

Stock Up

Fondos are designed to be scenic, which means they're usually somewhat remote. Course signage can be easy to miss, so have a plan if you get lost. Bring a course map, phone, cash, and a multi-tool.

Prepare to Share

If you're gunning for speed, slipping into a group will help you save energy. But don't wait

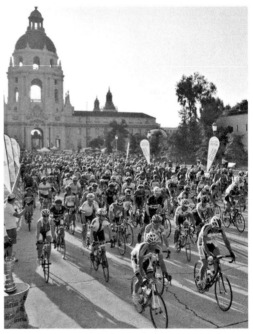

Riders at the start of the Gran Fondo Giro d'Italia in Los Angeles.

for event day to try it for the first time. Build group rides into your training to practice sticking close to someone else's wheel.

Start Smart

Thousands of riders will line up together, the faster ones in positions closer to the front. Rolling out with the right crowd is crucial if you take the competition seriously. Starting farther back may protect you from the chaos. Not sure where you should be? See the "Survive the Mass Start" below.

Meter Your Effort

A fondo might be a race against the clock, but it's no time trial. Drafting isn't cheating—it's strategy. Work with other riders to keep the pace high on flat sections, but save your hardest efforts for the timed climbs. "The classic mistake is taking it minute by minute instead of as a whole," says Cannondale/Cyclocrossworld.com pro cyclist Tim Johnson. At the L'Étape du California, the Tour of California's gran fondo, Johnson has seen overeager riders kill themselves early to stay

SURVIVE THE MASS START

MANAGE THE CHAOS WITH THESE THREE STRATEGIES.

KNOW YOUR PLACE

MOST FONDOS START PROS AND LICENSED RACERS up front, with casual riders behind them. "If you're unsure or intimidated, start closer to the back," advises Hunter Ziesing of team Hammer Nutrition/Charity of Choice. He also suggests joining a few group rides beforehand if you've never ridden en masse.

STAKE OUT YOUR TERRITORY

ONCE YOU LOCATE A SPOT, STAND NEXT to your bike to buy extra elbow room. A minute or two before the start, swing a leg over your saddle and prepare to ride. Make sure your helmet is buckled, your shoes are secure, and your bike is in the right gear to pedal as soon as the pack surges forward.

FIND YOUR FLOW

IF YOU'RE NOT STARTING AT THE FRONT, don't try to gun it out of the gate, says Ziesing. Stuck in a hard-charging pack? Maintain a comfortable speed and drift to the right. Then, without slamming on your brakes and causing a pileup, let speedier riders pass.

with the elite guys, then pop when it counted—on the 4.3-mile climb at 9 percent up Mt. Baldy.

Stack Your Deck

If the event ranks results by age, join forces with riders in various age groups, which preserves everyone's incentive to work together.

24 HOURS OF GRAN FONDO

Follow this timeline to make your big ride go smoothly.

The Day Before

4 P.M.: Have your bike clean and ready: race number attached, chain lubed, bolts tightened, tires fresh and topped off. Your seat bag should contain a mini-tool, spare tube or patches, and CO_2 cartridges (or carry a frame pump).

6 P.M.: Eat a balanced dinner that emphasizes carbs. Choose foods that agree with you; don't overdo it.

9 P.M.: Affix race number to jersey. Fill drink bottles and refrigerate. Lay out clothing and your gear: cell phone, cash, credit card, ID, wind/rain jacket or vest, on-bike snacks. Consider bringing an old sweater or garbage bag you can ditch before the start in case of bad weather.

Race Day

5 A.M. (OR WAKE-UP TIME): Aim for 400 to 800 calories at breakfast, mostly carbs and easy-to-digest protein, says Monique Ryan, RD, author of *Sports Nutrition for Endurance Athletes*. Good options include two slices of whole grain bread with peanut butter or oatmeal with fruit and nuts. Have your regular tea or coffee plus a few glasses of water.

6:30 A.M. (30 MINUTES TO START): Get to your corral about 30 minutes before the start (earlier for events with 3,000-plus riders). Top off your tank with a bar, gel, or even a banana right before the start.

7:00 A.M. (START TIME): Don't bother jostling to the front; most events segment riders based on estimated finish time. Take it leisurely. You're in for a long day.

7:30 A.M.: Start drinking a half hour after you roll, says Ryan. Water is good, but energy drinks provide fluids, electrolytes, and calories. Aim for 4 to 8 ounces every 15 to 20 minutes. Graze at aid stations: a banana, a cookie, something salty.

RIDE LIKE AN ITALIAN

LOOKING FOR A FONDO NEAR YOU? Go to Bicycling.com/eventfinder.

4:00 P.M.: Celebrate with food and drink at the finish. Hang out at the awards ceremony to score your competition or raffle prize. Start planning your next gran fondo.

Pro Tip

DON'T TAKE IT TOO SERIOUSLY. The cool part of a fondo, says veteran racer Tim Johnson, is that you can push as hard as you like or enjoy yourself as much as you want. "If you want to go for it and absolutely tap yourself out physically, it's a safe environment to do that," he says. But with thousands of like-minded cyclists on the course and a full support staff, it's also the perfect opportunity to simply enjoy a great day on your bike.

GRAN FONDO TRAINING PLAN

Ready to tackle a gran fondo? This 8-week plan focuses on building endurance and improving pedaling efficiency so you can finish an event of 100 miles with enough energy left over to enjoy the post-ride festivities. Total weekly riding time builds from 6 hours to 9.5 hours and includes one long ride on the weekend; you'll also enjoy two complete rest days per week. Before attempting this plan, you should already have several weeks of low-intensity riding under your belt (riding 4 to 5 times a week at an easy effort for 60 to 90 minutes).

Workouts

ACTIVE RECOVERY: Easy gear and no hard efforts.

ENDURANCE (END): Focus on a steady effort that you can maintain over a long duration and still finish strong. Your effort should pick up slightly on the hills and recover on the descents. This ride will develop the endurance you need to complete an event in the 100-mile range.

GROUP RIDE: The goal of doing a group ride is to get used to riding in close proximity with others and to the harder efforts required to keep up with a pack. Local cycling clubs will often offer an intro ride for first-time riders. Clubs are listed by region at usacycling.org. More experienced riders who have ridden with a group before should hop into a local Saturday ride and push beyond their usual pace.

HILL WORK: Choose a hill that takes at least 5 minutes to climb; make note of your location at the end of 5 minutes. Each time up, aim to reach the same point or farther. Do your hard efforts slightly above threshold pace (roughly equivalent to the maximum effort you can maintain over an hour of riding) at the easiest cadence possible. Finish the final repeat tired but with the ability to do one more. This will ensure that your pacing is correct and that your effort is being evenly distributed over the set of intervals.

TECHNIQUE WORK: Keep your effort low to moderate; the goal is to work on quality and to hit the cadence targets. Stay seated during these intervals. If you have trouble hitting the recommended cadence without bouncing out of the saddle, take it as high as possible without bouncing. During the single-leg drills, the goal is to make smooth, round pedal strokes for a minute with only one foot clipped in at a time. After the minute is up, switch sides and work the other leg. Try not to tense up or rotate your pelvis back. These drills are easiest to do on an indoor trainer. Exercise caution on the road and be sure that you can handle the bike with one foot unclipped (riding on flat terrain is best). Don't worry if you can't complete the entire minute in the first few weeks; aim to increase your time by 5 to 10 seconds each session, until you reach 1 minute.

TEMPO: Tempo workouts accomplish a lot of work in a short amount of time, improving both your endurance and threshold power. On these intervals, aim for about 10 percent below your threshold pace. That means you'll feel like you're working hard, but you should never be at your max. One way to gauge your effort: You should be able to have a choppy conversation with a riding partner. When training outside, short pauses for traffic lights and intersections are fine.

Ready to not just survive a gran fondo, but conquer it? Download our advanced plan at Bicycling.com/grandfondotraining.

Gran Fondo Training Plan

WEEK	MONDAY	TUESDAY	
1	Rest day	**Hill work** 1hr **END** with 4 × [4 min hard climbing + 5 min recovery] 1 hr	
2	Rest day	**Hill work** **END** with 4 × [5 min hard climbing + 5 min recovery] 1 hr	
3	Rest day	**Hill work** **END** with 5 × [5 min hard climbing + 5 min recovery] 1 hr	
4	Rest day	**Active recovery ride** 1 hr	
5	Rest day	**Hill work** **END** with 4 × [5 min hard-effort climbing, seated at 70 rpm + 5 min recovery] 1 hr	
6	Rest day	**Hill work** **END** with 4 × [5 min hard-effort climbing, seated at 65 rpm + 5 min recovery] 1 hr	
7	Rest day	**Hill work** **END** with 4 × [5 min hard-effort climbing, seated at 60 rpm + 5 min recovery] 1 hr	
8	Rest day	**Active recovery ride** 1 hr	

	WEDNESDAY	THURSDAY	FRIDAY	SATURDAY	SUNDAY
	Technique work **END** with 2 × [5 min high cadence at 105–110 rpm + 5 min recovery] 2 × 1 min single-leg pedaling each side 1 hr	**END** with 2 × [12 min Tempo effort + 5 min recovery] 1 hr	Rest day	**Group ride** 1 hr, 15 min or **END** with 2 × [12 min alternating hard effort and recovery every minute]. Recover at an easy effort for 10 min after each 12-min interval. 1 hr, 15 min	**END** 2 hr
	Technique work **END** with 2 × [8 min high cadence at 105–110 rpm + 5 min recovery] 3 × 1 min single-leg pedaling each side 1 hr	**END** with 2 × [15 min Tempo effort + 5 min recovery] 1 hr	Rest day	**Group ride** 1 hr, 30 min or **END** with 2 × [16 min alternating hard effort and recovery every minute]. Recover at an easy effort for 10 min after each 16-min interval. 1 hr, 30 min	**END** 2 hr, 30 min
	Technique work **END** with 2 × [10 min high cadence at 105–110 rpm + 5 min recovery] 4 × 1 min single-leg pedaling each side 1 hr	**END** with 2 × [20 min Tempo effort + 5 min recovery] 1 hr	Rest day	**Group ride** 1 hr, 30 min or **END** with 2 × [20 min alternating hard effort and recovery every minute]. Recover at an easy effort for 10 min after each 20-min interval. 1 hr, 30 min	**END** 3 hr
	Active recovery ride 1 hr	**END** with 2 × [8 min Tempo effort + 5 min recovery] 1 hr	Rest day	**Group ride** 1 hr or **END** with 2 × [5 min high cadence at 115–120 rpm + 5 min recovery between efforts] 4 × 1 min single-leg pedaling each side 1 hr	**END** 3 hr, 30 min
	Technique work **END** with 2 × [8 min high cadence at 115–120 rpm + 5 min recovery] 4 × 1 min single-leg pedaling each side 1 hr	**END** with 2 × [20 min Tempo effort + 5 min recovery] 1 hr	Rest day	**Group ride** 1 hr or **END** with 2 × [12 min alternating hard effort and recovery every minute]. Recover at an easy effort for 10 min after each 12-min interval. 1 hr	**END** with 20 min Tempo effort 4 hr
	Technique work **END** with 2 × [10 min high cadence at 115–120 rpm + 5 min recovery] 4 × 1 min single-leg pedaling each side 1 hr	Tempo **END** with 2 × [20 min Tempo effort + 5 min recovery] 1 hr	Rest day	**Group ride** 1 hr, 30 min or **END** with 2 × [18 min alternating hard effort and recovery every minute]. Recover at an easy effort for 10 min after each 18-min interval. 1 hr, 30 min	**END** with 30 min Tempo effort 4 hr
	Technique work **END** with 2 × [10 min high cadence at 115–120 rpm + 5 min recovery] 4 x 1 min single-leg pedaling each side 1 hr	**END** with 2 × [20 min Tempo effort + 5 min recovery] 1 hr	Rest day	**Group ride** 1 hr, 30 min or **END** with 2 × [20 min alternating hard effort and recovery every minute]. Recover at an easy effort for 10 min after each 20-min interval. 1 hr, 30 min	**END** with 30 min Tempo effort 4 hr, 30 min
	Active recovery ride 1 hr	**END** with 2 × [10 min Tempo effort+ 5 min recovery] 1 hr	Travel day 30–60 min Active recovery	Option 1: Saturday Gran Fondo Event Option 2: Travel day 30–60 min Active recovery Option 3: Leg-opener workout [if event is on Sunday] 2 × [3 min ramp-up to Threshold + 2 min hold at Threshold + 5 min recovery effort] and 2 × [10-sec sprints out of the saddle + 2 min recovery]	Sunday Gran Fondo Event

PART IV

COMPETE

Once you've got group-riding basics down and lots of miles under your belt, consider increasing the stakes with some sanctioned racing. From registration to number pinning, we'll take all the intimidation out of getting started. From there you can choose your poison—road, cyclocross, and cross-country mountain bike races are all demystified inside.

CHAPTER 10

Racing 101

There's a feeling that you can get only from racing and finishing—
the feeling of pushing yourself beyond what you're capable of
doing in training. It's about achieving the ultimate physical
accomplishment—and you can't feel that on the sidelines.

—NED OVEREND, US PROFESSIONAL CROSS-COUNTRY
MOUNTAIN BIKE RACER, FORMER WORLD CHAMPION,
AND MULTI-TIME NATIONAL CHAMPION

BIKE RACING IS LIKELY TO BE DIFFERENT THAN ANY OTHER
sport you've competed in. If you have a background in running or triathlons, don't
expect to be able to set your internal cruise control to a sustainable pace and breeze
in to the finish. Likewise, mentally zoning out or slowing down to enjoy the scenery
is usually out of the question. While it's true that the intensity of competitions usually
ebb and flow, one thing every experienced rider will tell you is that bike racing is
about suffering. How long can you put yourself in the pain cave and stay there? How
many repeat efforts can you make going full gas? During races your legs will burn
more than you ever thought possible on a bike.

Victories don't always go to the rider who's strongest, however. Sometimes the spoils are scooped up by the smartest. After your brain adapts to riding in close quarters, you learn to expend mental energy not only reading the course but also reading your competitors. Strategy and tactics come into play. It's like trying to play a chess match while you run a marathon. It's challenging and stimulating and frustrating in ways you may not have experienced in other athletic endeavors. But it's also rewarding. This chapter will prepare you for that journey.

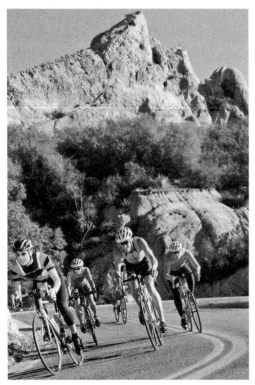

Number-one rule: Keep the rubber side down.

What Kind of Race Should You Do?

TIME TRIAL

WHAT IT IS: The classic race against the clock; no drafting, no tactics. May the best sufferer win.

DO IT IF: You're not ready to embrace the complexity of racing in a group.

KEY TERM: *Aero.* Short for "aerodynamic"— a concept you'll try to explain to your family when they ask why you spent $1,800 on wheels.

ONE-DAY ROAD RACE

WHAT IT IS: A competition that can be flat and cobbled, paved and hilly, or anything in between; rewards riders possessing endurance and the tactical smarts to conserve energy.

DO IT IF: Your friends frequently beg you to stop hammering during the last 10 miles of a century.

KEY TERM: *Feed zone.* The place where your significant other will stand all day, waiting to hand you a bottle—and then watch in horror as you drop it while riding away.

CRITERIUM

WHAT IT IS: The most popular race in America, a "crit" provides nonstop, NASCAR-style action as riders hit the gas for 20 laps or more on a closed, often technical course usually less than a mile long. See where the spectators are standing? That's where you're most likely to go down.

DO IT IF: You're a good bike handler looking for a thrill and don't mind patching road rash.

KEY TERM: *Prime* (rhymes with "team"). A prize for winning a lap—or a good excuse to end your race early by sprinting for a bike shop gift certificate. When someone asks how your day went, say you won $20 and leave it at that.

STAGE RACE

WHAT IT IS: A multiday event that typically has something for everyone. Expect a time trial, a road race with some climbing, and a criterium.

DO IT IF: You're a solid all-around rider with plenty of vacation days to burn.

KEY TERM: *Leader's jersey.* Bestowed upon the racer with the lowest overall time, it might as well have a target on the back. It's difficult to keep if you don't have teammates to help you defend it.

MOUNTAIN BIKE–CROSS COUNTRY

WHAT IT IS: An off-road discipline that requires high levels of skill and coordination. Expect conditions that range from packed dirt to hilly trails riddled with rocks and roots.

DO IT IF: You're looking for a low-key, friendly scene.

KEY TERM: *Singletrack.* A narrow mountain bike trail that must be ridden single file.

CYCLOCROSS

WHAT IT IS: A mix of road and mountain biking with some running and stair climbing thrown in for good measure. The season typically runs through the fall and winter.

DO IT IF: You want to have a blast while improving your bike-handling skills or you have lots of thermal underwear and nothing better to do.

KEY TERM: *Hand-ups.* This is the practice of spectators holding out incentives for riders to try to grab—everything from beer to bacon to

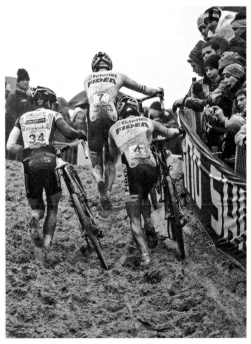

If you like getting dirty, you'll love 'cross.

cold hard cash. However, for USA Cycling–sanctioned races (see below), hand-ups may be illegal or restricted to a designated zone. Be sure to ask beforehand so you don't get disqualified.

Get Registered

USA Cycling is the main governing body for bike racing in the United States. It's comprised of more than 2,500 clubs and teams and 75,303 licensees, which include officials, coaches, mechanics, race directors, and competitive cyclists of all ages and abilities across all five disciplines of the sport. Nearly 3,000 competitive and noncompetitive cycling events each year are sanctioned by USA Cycling. If you want to compete in USA Cycling–sanctioned races you'll need a racing license from USA Cycling (usacycling.org). Beginners can buy a one-day license online (or sometimes at the event) for $15 ($10 for mountain bike). If you plan on racing multiple times, or just want to take advantage of the discounts and insurance offered to members, you should buy an annual license for $70. Cyclists are divided into categories according to ability and experience, with separate races for each group. For instance, men who race on the road begin as a Category 5 rider and earn upgrade points at first just by competing in races and, once in higher categories, by placing. Results count toward upgrades all the way to Category 1, the highly competitive top of the amateur food chain. Download the free USA Cycling app, My USAC, to find and register for races, track your license information, and view your results.

Find a Race in Your Backyard

USA Cycling is a great resource for their approved races, but it's not your only bet. Regional racing associations are on the rise. To find a race near you, check online for associations in for your region. See below for a short list of some regional groups and their web sites. And, from the obvious-but-necessary file, ask at your local bike shop: In many towns (and almost every city), there are weekly low-key, after-work races that offer a cheap and relatively stress-free way to get your tires wet.

- California Bicycle Racing, californiabicycleracing.org: California road racing
- Eastern Fat Tire Association, efta.com: New England mountain biking
- American Bicycle Racing, ambikerace.com: Midwest road racing
- Bicycle Racing Association of Colorado, coloradocycling.org: mountain, cyclocross, and road racing
- Oregon Bicycle Racing Association, obra.org: Oregon mountain and road biking

Signing Your Life Away?

Legal waivers are a necessary part of organized rides—but they don't apply to every mishap.

If you've ever participated in an organized ride or race, you probably signed a release—a document that protects the event organizer from liability for negligence if you are injured or killed or if your bike is damaged. You're typically required to sign the release before you're allowed to participate.

This situation creates a conundrum for cyclists. By signing, you're agreeing to waive some legal rights in the event of injury. On the other hand, without liability releases there would be few such events because organizers wouldn't want to assume the legal risk of holding one. When asked, I usually recommend organizers require signed waivers.

What if something goes wrong and you are injured? Signing the release doesn't mean you have no recourse if someone else is at fault. Your options vary depending on what happened and the ride's location.

First of all, any participants not named in the release may be held liable if they played a part in your injury. The parties named in the release are protected, but not from liability for gross or criminal negligence, recklessness, or intentional acts—like if an event volunteer

WAIVER BASICS

WHO CAN'T SIGN

IF A RIDER IS YOUNGER THAN 18, his signature on a contract is unenforceable. As for parents who sign a waiver on the child's behalf? That signature is no more legally binding than the child's.

WHO IS PROTECTED

THE PEOPLE AND PARTIES NAMED IN THE release. This typically includes event organizers, officials and volunteers, event sponsors, medical personnel, relevant governmental entities, and participating clubs. Some releases may include other riders as well.

WHO ISN'T PROTECTED

ANY PARTY NOT NAMED. IF ANOTHER RIDER not mentioned in the waiver or a driver on an open course causes you to crash, you may have legal rights against those parties.

does something so reckless that it is almost inevitable riders will be injured.

Even if something unforeseeable happened—for example, a car appeared on a closed course—the release may not protect organizers against the ordinary negligence of a volunteer allowing the car into the ride. And if organizers proffer a release that claims to shield them against liability for all acts, don't worry: Courts have shot down releases claiming such all-encompassing coverage.

In some jurisdictions, releases are essentially worthless. This is because some officials believe as a matter of public policy that letting people escape liability for negligence is a bad idea. So if you get hurt on an organized ride, don't assume you're stuck with the tab.

Race Prep

Some of this is going to sound obvious, but after you leave your front wheel in the driveway, your shoes on top of your car, and your shorts on the kitchen table, you understand the power of the obvious. Here are the five most crucial rules of getting race ready.

1. Don't overhaul your drivetrain the night before a race, or you'll almost surely suffer skipping gears as cables stretch. In fact, don't do anything major to your bike the day before a race, unless a crisis forces your hand.

2. Do go over your bike with hex wrenches to ensure everything is appropriately snug. Pay particular attention to the brake pads.

3. Don't eat anything weird the day before. Or, if all you eat is weird, don't eat anything normal. Point being, don't mess with your diet.

Pro Tip
Don't take the day off before a big event. If you need complete rest from riding, do so 2 days before, then take a short ride on the eve of the event—including a couple sprints to make sure your body (and your bike) are well oiled.

4. Don't wait to pack your bag until race morning. Pack it the night before and go through it again in the morning. I like to keep a bag packed with all the nonperishables in the closet. Make sure you have these in your bag: a change of clothes, your race outfit (including helmet), a towel, enough water to rinse off with and to drink, water bottles filled with your competition drink of choice, race food, recovery food (and lots of it), sunscreen and sunglasses, flip-flops for post-race BS-ing, and your race license.

In cool/rainy weather, add a thermos of tea, a knit hat, and a waterproof shell to your bag.

5. Small luxuries can salvage a rough day. Consider packing some of these: a cooler packed with beer and sandwiches (for after the race), solar shower (the height of racing savvy, particularly among the mountain bike crowd, who won't mind when you strip naked in the parking lot), camp chair, work stand, fully stocked toolbox, and first aid kit.

Pro Tip

Know your gear. "Don't ever use anything new in a bike race," says former pro racer and cycling commentator Frankie Andreu. This advice applies to backcountry mountain bike rides, charity events, or exotic cycling vacations. Log some miles on fresh equipment before embarking on any serious ride. You don't want to be 60 miles from home when you discover that you and your new saddle aren't soul mates after all.

Style Tips

Just because you're a newbie doesn't mean you have to look like one. Here are 12 ways to fake it 'til you make it.

1. For road races, take off your saddlebag to save weight and show the proper laissez-faire attitude toward breakdowns. For a mountain bike race: If your bench grinder fits into your hydration pack, take it.

2. When you realize your front brake is squealing during warm-ups, do not stop to adjust it. Pedal casually to the nearest car, hide behind it, and do the repair. In public, your bike must be impeccable.

3. When registering, don't ask if the officials have safety pins. (They do, in a box right there on the table. Look.) And don't ask, "Where do I put my number?" Display confidence with a question that implies familiarity—"Number on the side, right?"—and which will, when corrected, elicit the information you need.

4. Don't drive to the race in your bike clothes. Wear civvies. Never change in the portable toilet or while squiggling like a pervert in the front seat of your car. Better to discreetly drop trou while facing the open door of your car. Don't fret the backside—everyone's used to seeing booty at a race.

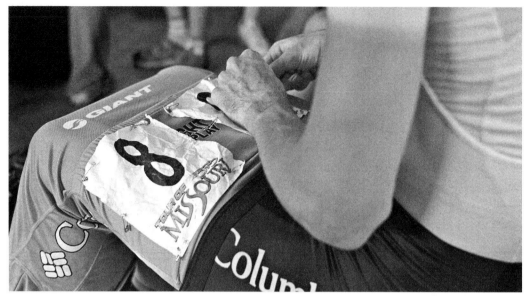

Eight is great but fewer pins work, too.

5. Pee the first time you have to. Ignore the next three urges, then indulge your bladder one last time. Never pee more than five times.

6. Pin your number correctly. Here's how.

- If you attach your number before you kit up, stretch your jersey across your lap to mimic the shape of your body. A pillow works, too, if used at home—in public, the dork factor is high.

- Ignore any prepunched holes in the corners. Instead, make two holes with each pin: one to go down through the number and jersey and another to come back up and out.

- The cool kids crumple their race numbers to keep them from parachuting—but technically, that could get you disqualified. Remember: You can use more than four pins.

7. Beware the "cat 5 tattoo." Remove chainring marks from your calves before lining up.

8. Avoid yelling "Hold your line!" at everybody who gets in your way. Don't be that person.

9. Don't throw empty food wrappers onto the course. Stuff them in your jersey pockets.

10. Don't don another team's clothing. Save the BMC kit for your training ride.

11. Sprinting for a nonresult is a no-no. Etiquette dictates that you coast in if you're outside the top 10 or the points or prize list.

12. Don't post a victory salute for any result other than the win, including midrace sprints.

Warm-Up Rules

WHAT IT IS: A short effort before a ride or race.

WHAT IT DOES: Preps your body to work hard. It helps your muscles contract faster, and you can sustain a higher heart rate. Blood flow also speeds up, delivering fuel to and removing waste from muscles faster.

WHEN AND HOW MUCH: It depends on the event. For a long road race, you might do a shorter one or use the first 10 miles as the warm-up. For a time trial or hill climb, in which you need to go all-out from the start, get in a 30- to 45-minute warm-up beforehand.

7

Number of seconds faster cyclists rode a 3-kilometer time trial after warming up, versus when they did the time trial cold.

STICK TO YOUR PLAN: Warm up too hard or for too long and you'll dip into precious energy stores, says Hunter Allen, founder of Peaks Coaching Group and coauthor of *Cutting-Edge Cycling*. Cut it short and you may struggle at the beginning of your event.

TAKE 10: Aim to finish warming up about 10 minutes before it's go time, says Allen.

ADJUST FOR WEATHER: On a chilly day, it's okay to warm up for longer or time it so you finish closer to the event start. In hot weather, keep it minimal. Your muscles will heat up quickly. The longer your event is, the shorter your warm-up should be.

Try these sample warm-ups from Allen.

EVENT	WARM-UP
Criterium Time trial Cyclocross	20 minutes easy, 4 × [1 minute fast pedaling at 120 rpms + 1 minute easy], 5 minutes all-out, 5 minutes easy
Road race <60 miles	10–15 minutes easy, 5 × [1–2 minutes at 85 percent race pace + 2–3 minutes recovery], 5 minutes easy
Road race >60 miles	10–15 minutes easy, 5 minutes tempo [about 80 percent race pace], 5 minutes easy
Ultraendurance events >5 hours	10 minutes easy pedaling as you roll out from the start

The Razor's Edge: Why Shave

Neither specific historical reference nor objective scientific finding can account for why male cyclists shave their legs, but here are the most-cited reasons.

IT IMPROVES YOUR AERODYNAMICS ON THE BIKE. In this age of seamless skinsuits, aero frames, dimpled helmets, and ultralight deep-rim carbon wheels, it's senseless to ignore the slight but real advantage of having bare legs. (To wit, a 1987 study conducted by biomechanical engineer Chester Kyle for *Bicycling* magazine concluded that the aerodynamic improvement is roughly 0.6 percent, which could result in a savings of around 5 seconds in a 40-K time trial ridden at 37 kilometers per mile. Interestingly, Specialized recently retested this and found it saves an average of 70 seconds over a 40-K time trial.)

IT IMPROVES THE BENEFITS AND PLEASURE OF MASSAGE. Getting your hair pulled during massage hurts. A lot.

IT MAKES WOUND CARE EASIER AND MORE EFFECTIVE. Cleaning and caring for road rash is simpler and heals faster when there's no leg hair present to impede the removal of dirt and grime, host bacteria, or complicate bandage changes.

IT JUST LOOKS BETTER—AND THAT MAKES YOU FASTER. Every cut and line of toned muscles pop when not obscured by a thicket of hair, and the snazzier you look, the sharper you ride.

IT'S TRADITION. Losing the leg pelt is a sign that you're committed to living your life with the noble aim of honoring what it means to be a true racing cyclist—plus, showing up hairy to a serious group ride is akin to wearing shorts to church.

CHAPTER 11

Road Races

Cycling in general, and racing in particular, has a way of ordering and fulfilling our lives. When we get into cycling, we inherit a point of view, a perception, an attitude toward life.

—OWEN MULHOLLAND, CYCLING WRITER

SPEED, SUFFERING, STRATEGY, RISK—SKINNY-TIRE COMPETI-tions have it all. This chapter encompasses the types of road races you'll probably need a USA Cycling license for: one-day races, crits, and time trials. Whether you want to pick one big event to target for the year or enter multiple races between March and September (sign up for a stage race and you'll do all three in a weekend!), we've got the info you need. Read on for race-specific training plans as well as tips and tricks for mastering each discipline.

One-Day Road Race

The road race is a mass-start, one-day event. The courses may be long or short, flat or hilly, or a combination. A road race is rarely a contest of who can pedal the hardest. It's more of a pulse-pounding game of psychology, skill, and luck. The athlete with the greatest overall ability to sprint, climb, and just persevere will tend to have the most success. While you shouldn't expect to win your first time out, you should try to navigate the event with the savvy of a more experienced rider—both on and off the course. Here's your guide.

BEFORE

Check in, pin on your number, and prep your bike. Then, about 30 minutes before the start, get in a quick spin to warm up. Use the time to locate the mechanic's pit or support vehicles, first-aid tent, and precise location of the finish line. (*Important*: Wear your helmet—it's a rule.) Get to the starting line at least 10 minutes before go time and listen closely to prerace instructions specific to the event and course.

DURING

There's no need for a furious start—allow a group to form in front of you, then draft among or behind them. The idea is to keep up while pedaling as little as possible. Prevent a gap from opening between you and riders ahead, which will help you save energy so you can pass dropped riders or stay with the leaders over hills. Above all, relax. Races play out in one of two ways: Either a small group accelerates away from the main field and those riders duke it out among themselves, or the entire group stays together and gallops to the line. Increase your odds of making the winning breakaway by riding aggressively when others are tired—on climbs or after fast sections. If a field sprint

DOS AND DON'TS OF RACE SAFETY

DO	DON'T
➤ Hold a steady line through corners	➤ Slow abruptly or jam on the brakes
➤ Communicate road hazards to riders nearby	➤ Make erratic movements (but you should always expect others to do so)
➤ Watch body language to anticipate where other riders might go	➤ Stop or swerve after the finish line

looks like a possibility, position yourself near the front of the group but stay out of the wind until the final 100 to 200 meters, when you can unleash an all-out charge to the finish.

AFTER

Race officials typically post results near the registration area. Standings become final after a 15-minute protest period. Earned a prize? Collect it by presenting your race number and license at the registration table.

HOW TO BREAK AWAY

The act of escaping the clutches of the pack is one of the misunderstood tactical arts of competitive cycling: The escapist is not faster than everyone in the pack and certainly not speedier than the collective power of the pack. He is simply one who understands how to exploit the group's moments of weakness or inattention and, once away, can stay calm enough to manage the gap through the various chases and lulls that are sure to follow. And he can also suffer like Prometheus.

1. **PICK YOUR MOMENT.** The most common mistake inexperienced riders make is to attack when they feel strong. A better strategy is to attack when everyone else feels weak—the key to getting away is not how fast you can go, but the difference between your speed and the pack's. Likewise, sometimes the best place to attack is not the base of a climb but just as the group comes over a peak, when many cyclists often inadvertently relax because they assume the big effort is over. Another good spot is on a twisty road, where you can quickly get out of sight around a bend.

2. **DON'T LOOK BACK, BUT DON'T BE A SUCKER.** When you attack, try to project the idea that you have no doubt you'll ride away from everyone. A cyclist who peeks backward appears to be anticipating capture. On the other hand, don't plow blindly ahead while a chase group sits in your draft (it's happened to some good riders) or burn yourself to a nub just ahead of a group riding comfortably while keeping you within easy catching distance. Listen for clues that riders are close, look sideways for shadows, sneak a peripheral glance on turns. If you don't feel you've escaped, you haven't. Sit up, let the group catch you, then attack again.

3. **COOPERATE.** If you attack and others go with you, form a smooth paceline as soon as you can. It's customary to allow riders who bridged a little time to recover; let them skip a few turns at the front, then insist they share the work. (If they won't, attack again to shed them.) If there is a known end point—like a town sign—agree among yourselves how close to the line you will work together to stave off the chasing pack. At some point you will have to attack each other to try to win, but until then, you

want to eliminate all high jinks and share the sole goal of staying away.

TRAINING PLAN

The road races can consist of 5- to 25-mile repeating loops, starting and finishing at the same point. The courses may vary in terrain; some contain a mix of elevations, others are predominately flat. The athlete with the greatest overall ability to sprint, climb, and just persevere will tend to have the most success, so your training plan needs to support this.

This plan is for the road cyclist who wants to do a road race and has between 7 to 12 hours a week to train. Before you start it, you should have 4 to 6 weeks of "base" training totaling at least 500 miles of riding under your belt. The plan consists of workouts at various effort levels. It offers wattage, heart rate, and rate of perceived exertion options so you can gauge your effort whether you use a power meter, a heart rate monitor, or prefer to work out by feel.

To really finish strong, you need to put in some hard efforts. As James Herrera, MS, expert cycling coach and founder of Performance Driven in Colorado Springs, Colorado, points out, a successful race training plan means building volume *and* intensity—and this plan definitely does both. *Note:* This plan requires some very hard efforts, which means you need to listen to your body. If you're feel-

ing drained, overtired, or unprepared for your next ride, take an extra rest day to recover.

Workouts

GROUP RIDE—AGGRESSIVE: During your group ride, look to complete the following: Make five aggressive attacks with full-power attack sprints and stay off the front for at least 1 to 2 minutes, bridge two to three gaps of another rider (great to do from back of pack), climb three short hills at best efforts, and look to take a long functional threshold power level pull for 10 minutes (or sit in wind). Finally, have fun in the race for home and look for ways to "win"—make the break, look to attack, or outsprint them at the town line.

MAX VO$_2$ MICRO INTERVALS: This is an interval where you vary effort from 30 seconds in zone 6 to zone 1 for the duration of the intervals.

MAX VO$_2$ BUILDERS: Find a course with three to five longer hill climbs. Start out in zone 2 and with each climb put in a 3-to-5-minute effort in zone 5. After each effort, ride at low endurance for at least 5 minutes to recover then go back up to the prescribed endurance zone. Cadence: 85 to 105.

BURSTS: Ride in zone 2. Vary your cadence throughout the ride and work on your pedaling form. Practice "coming over the top" and "pulling through the bottom" of the pedal (pretend there is glass in your shoes). Cadence: 85 to 105.

Road Race Training Plan

WEEK	MONDAY	TUESDAY	WEDNESDAY	THURSDAY	FRIDAY	SATURDAY	SUNDAY
1	Rest day	**END** with 30 min Tempo 1 hr, 30 min	**END** with 3 × 5 min Max VO_2 micro intervals (zone 5); 5 min rest 1 hr, 15 min	**END** with 3 × 8 Max VO_2 micro intervals; 5 min rest in zone 2 1 hr, 15 min	**Active recovery** 1 hr	**END** with Max VO_2 builders 2 hr, 15 min Note: It's okay to go longer today! If you want, you can do 3–4 hours, but not too much more than you are used to. **ALTERNATE WORKOUT:** Group ride—aggressive	**END** with Bursts 2 hr, 15 min

Total hours: 9:30:00

WEEK	MONDAY	TUESDAY	WEDNESDAY	THURSDAY	FRIDAY	SATURDAY	SUNDAY
2	Rest day	**END** with 5 × 1 min (zone 6); 2 min rest 1 hr	**END** 1 hr, 30 min	**END** with 4 × 5 min (zone 5); 5 min rest 1 hr, 30 min	**Active recovery** 1 hr	**END** with 30–40 min Tempo with 5 × 20 sec (zone 4) 2 hr, 30 min **ALTERNATE WORKOUT:** Group ride—aggressive	**END** with 2 × 12 min (zone 3.5); 5 min rest 2 hr, 30 min

Total hours: 10:00:00

WEEK	MONDAY	TUESDAY	WEDNESDAY	THURSDAY	FRIDAY	SATURDAY	SUNDAY
3	Rest day	**END** with 6 × 3 min (zone 5); 3 min rest 1 hr, 30 min	**END** with 30 min Tempo 1 hr, 30 min	**END** with 4 × 8 min Max VO_2 micro intervals; 5 min rest in zone 2 1 hr, 30 min	**Active recovery** 1 hr	**END** with Max VO_2 builders 2 hr **ALTERNATE WORKOUT:** Group ride—aggressive	**END** with Bursts 3 hr

Total hours: 10:30:00

WEEK	MONDAY	TUESDAY	WEDNESDAY	THURSDAY	FRIDAY	SATURDAY	SUNDAY
4	Rest day	Rest day	**END** with 1 × (5 × 1 min in zone 6; 2 min rest). Rest for 5–8 minutes in between sets. 1 hr Note: Go as hard as you can from 1 min on, as these are maximal intervals.	IF RACING SATURDAY: **Rest day** IF RACING SUNDAY: **END** with 3 × 3 min (zone 5); 3 min rest 1 hr, 30 min	IF RACING SATURDAY: **END** with 3 × 90 sec (zone 5); 5 min rest 1 hr IF RACING SUNDAY: **Rest day**	IF RACING SUNDAY: **END** with 3 × 90 sec (zone 5); 5 min rest 1 hr **OR RACE**	**RACE**

Total hours: 6:30:00

Abbreviations: END, endurance/zone 2; max VO_2, maximum VO_2/zone 5; tempo, zone 3.

Criteriums

If watching the pros go for grand tour glory has revved up your competitive spirit, try a criterium. "These simple road races are the perfect way for new competitors to get their feet wet and improve fitness," says Michael Carter, an assistant director at Team Type 1. A criterium, or crit, is a bike race held on a short course (often on blocked-off city streets). The course is short, usually less than 5 km, and is a closed circuit where riders complete multiple laps. Riders typically race for a given length of time, then complete a specified number of laps. An example would be a race of 60 minutes plus three laps.

In addition to the typical method of determining a winner—first rider across the finish line—many crits have prizes that can be won while the race is in progress. Called *primes* (pronounced "preems"), these are given for winning specific laps along the way and are frequently cash prizes or merchandise. Criteriums are especially spectator-friendly, as the riders pass by a given point many times over the course of a race.

You don't need to be a hammer or king of

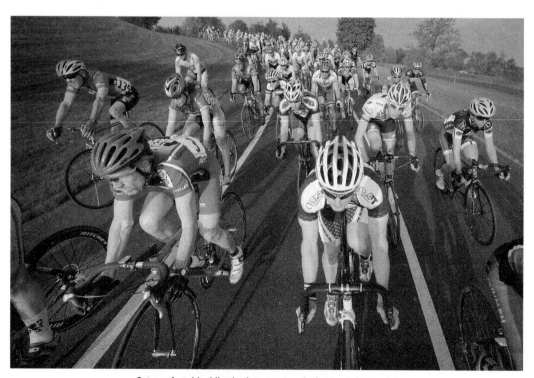

Get comfortable riding in close quarters before entering a crit.

the shop ride—anyone with a road bike and a helmet can enter a Category 5 race. Check Bicycling.com/eventfinder for a local crit and follow this advice so you finish your first race with a smile—if not a trophy.

CLOSE QUARTERS

Though racers technically shouldn't make contact in the pack, it happens often and a little preparation will help you avoid crashing. Join local group rides to build your pack-riding prowess, says Carter. For more practice, go to a grassy field with a friend and knock shoulders and handlebars at a low speed.

TRAIN FOR SPEED

Successful racers can sprint out of corners lap after lap and still have energy for the finish, says Frank Overton, owner of FasCat Coaching and a Level 1 USA Cycling coach. "Anaerobic intervals develop the power to match accelerations, attacks, and sprints," he says. He suggests doing this workout once a week: Warm up for 20 minutes, then perform four 1-minute intervals with a minute of recovery between each. When done, spin easy for 5 minutes, then repeat the set.

GET READY

If possible, ride the course before the race to get acquainted with its turns, rises, and descents. Then, if you have a stationary trainer or rollers, complete a 30-minute easy spin 45 minutes before the start, says Overton. Finish the warm-up with three 15-second sprint efforts to prepare your body for race intensity.

CARVE TURNS

"Focus on the curve's exit, not the wheel in front of you," Overton says. Keep your hands in the drops and place your weight on your outside pedal, with your foot in the 6 o'clock

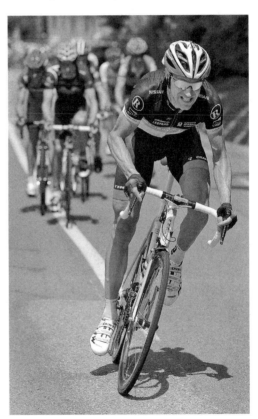

Be ready for multiple attacks.

position. "This lowers your center of gravity and increases stability," he says. If you feel uneasy, stay outside the pack on turns—you'll have more room to correct your line.

ATTACK THE PACK

There's no surefire way to predict whether a break will be successful, "but attacking when the peloton least expects it, or is just unwilling to chase, helps your odds," Carter says. Take off when another break is pulled back or in a strong headwind. If you're a climber, you can also surprise the bunch by attacking before— not on—a hill. If you're a strong sprinter, try surging ahead on a smaller climb. But, Carter adds, a break can succeed only if you strategize with other strong riders willing to work together; otherwise, you'll be back in the pack before you know it.

FINISH SMART

"Focus on the last lap," Overton says. "Get yourself into the top 10 and pedal hard through the last two turns." Start your sprint about 200 meters from the line and give it everything you have. Keep your hands in the drops and your head low to reduce wind drag. Don't go for it if you're not at the head of the pack, though. Sprinting for 13th place, Overton says, is how crashes happen.

INCREASE YOUR MENTAL TOUGHNESS

WHETHER YOU'RE RIDING A CRIT OR a road race, your brain can tire well before your body. "The mind can control so much of our experience on the bike," says Julie Browning, owner of Breakaway Training in Portland, Oregon. "Luckily, mental skills can be developed." She recommends trying these simple exercises during one ride a week to increase your focus and your chances for success during tough stretches.

During a rugged part of a ride, try counting pedal strokes. First, count three to five strokes on your right leg. This creates the illusion that the left leg isn't working as hard. Then do the same with your left, and then five pedal strokes without focusing on either leg. Repeat until you've moved into an easier part of the ride.

Another technique ideal for climbing: Count up to a predetermined number over and over again (1, 2, 3, 4; 1, 2, 3, 4) in time with your pedal strokes or try a two-syllable phrase such as "ticktock, ticktock." This helps you focus on the timing of your strokes rather than your suffering.

HOW TO WIN A SPRINT

At the club and recreational levels, even some of the most competent riders opt out of the fun because they're unsure what to do when the group sprints for the finish. Worse, some riders with more confidence than experience jump willy-nilly into the action, endangering everyone. Here's how to handle yourself in a bar-to-bar finish.

1. **BE PREDICTABLE.** On TV, or viewed from the back of an aggressive group, a sprint looks like an anything-goes melee in which the foolhardy triumph. In reality, although you need nerve to execute your plans—if you back out of a wind-sheltered hole in front of you, someone else will quickly pedal into it—good sprinters follow an accepted and predictable choreography that keeps the action as safe as possible. The etiquette can be complex, but most of the lessons can be simplified into one rule: Be smooth. Never perform an erratic maneuver. For instance, if a line of riders begins passing you, don't get excited and immediately swing over to try to join it. Instead, quickly glance back before you move to make sure you aren't riding into someone. Likewise, before you jump out of a line to make a dash for the finish, make sure you have a clear lane, with no one coming up fast behind you.

2. **HOLD YOUR LINE.** Don't angle across the road on a sprint, hoping to cut off or drop riders. (Pros are sometimes disqualified for extreme examples of this.) It's dangerous—because you're behaving unpredictably—and it's regarded as a bush-league tactic that reflects poorly on you. Also don't furiously rock your body; instead, with hands in the drops, rock the bike with each pedal stroke while your body stays centered.

3. **ACCELERATE WISELY.** The biggest mistake novices make in the final moments of a sprint is to swing out of a draft and try to accelerate into the wind. It's much smarter to let a slight gap open in front of you—about half a bike length—and begin accelerating toward the rider's wheel while you're still protected from the wind. Then when you swing out you will already be moving faster than the rider in front of you.

TRAINING PLAN

To succeed in crits, you need to be able to accelerate repeatedly and recover between efforts at higher speeds and intensities than you'd typically experience in long road races. This 4-week crit training plan is for the road cyclist who has between 7 and 12 hours a week to train. It will prepare you to ride in the pack, handle the speed, and be ready for the corners and hard jumps out of them, so you can go for the win. To ensure you are ready to complete this plan, you should have already completed 4 to 6 weeks of "base" training totaling at least 500 miles of riding. The plan consists of workouts at various effort levels. It offers wattage, heart rate, and rate of perceived exertion options so you can gauge your efforts whether you use a power meter or a heart rate monitor, or prefer to work out by feel.

Workouts

20/20 CRIT SPRINTS: To perform this set of crit sprints, you start from a slow roll, then jump hard out of the saddle with an explosive effort to get on top of the gear. When you have reached maximum cadence, sit down and maintain maximum intensity for the entire length of the effort, 20 pedal strokes. Then spin easy for 20 pedal strokes. Then jump hard, with maximum effort for 20 pedal strokes. Spin easy for 20 strokes. Repeat this process until you have completed the specified number of sprints. Perform these sprints on a flat to slightly uphill stretch of road or an indoor trainer. You will find that you need a long stretch of road for crit sprints. Keep that in mind when seeking out your training grounds. Gearing would be 53 × 16 or 53 × 14.

CRIT SPRINTS: Sprint as hard as you can from a high tempo speed for 10 seconds, then recover for a minute. Go for 20 seconds, with another minute recovery, and again for 30 seconds, and so on, until you get to 60 seconds

(obviously not sprinting, more a lead-out pace). After your 60-second interval take a 5-to-10-minute recovery (taking your bike for a walk), then go again. When you can't complete a full planned interval, STOP!

MAX VO$_2$ MICRO INTERVALS: During these intervals, vary your effort from 30 seconds in zone 6 to zone 1 for the duration of the intervals.

SST INTERVALS: Complete 2 x 12-minute intervals in the "Sweet Spot" (zone 3.5) with 5 minutes recovery in between. Ride all other time in level 2 endurance zone. Note: The sweet spot is a small area of intensity characterized by 88 to 93 percent of one's functional threshold power.

GROUP RIDE—AGGRESSIVE: Group rides can be helpful in our training as "mini-race" efforts as they often are fun, competitive, and create opportunity to build race skills. During your group ride, look to complete the following: make five aggressive attacks with full-power attack sprints and stay out front for at least 1 to 2 minutes, bridge two to three gaps of other rider (great to do from back of pack), climb three short hills at best efforts, and look to take a long functional threshold power level pull for 10 minutes (or sit in wind). Finally, have fun in the race for home and look for ways to "win"— make the break, look to attack, or outsprint them at the town line.

Criterium Training Plan

WEEK	MONDAY	TUESDAY	WEDNESDAY	THURSDAY	FRIDAY	SATURDAY	SUNDAY
1	Rest day	**END** with Tempo 1 hr END with 30 min zone 3	**END** with 2 × [5 × 1 min; 2 min rest]. Rest 5–8 minutes between sets. 1 hr Note: Go as hard as you can for the 1-min intervals.	**END** with 4 ×8 min Max VO$_2$ micro intervals; 5 min rest in zone 2 1 hr, 15 min	**Active recovery** 1 hr	**SST Intervals** 2 hr **Alternate Workout:** Group ride—aggressive	**END** 3 hr
Total hours: 9:30:00							
2	Rest day	**Crit sprints** 1 hr Note: Target completing 2 "sets"; go for 3 if feeling good!	**END** 1 hr, 30 min	**END** with Five 20/20 Crit sprints 1 hr, 30 min	**Active recovery** 1 hr	**END** 3 hr **Alternate Workout:** Group ride—aggressive	**END** with 4 × 8 min Micro intervals; 5 min rest in between in zone 2 2 hr
Total hours: 10:00:00							
3	Rest day	**END** with 3 × [5 × 1 min in zone 6; 2 min rest]. Rest 5–8 min between sets 1 hr, 15 min	**END** with 45 min zone 3 1 hr, 30 min	**Crit sprints** 1 hr, 15 min Target completing 3 "sets"; go for 4 if feeling good!	**Active recovery** 1 hr	**END** with 4 ×8 min Max VO$_2$ micro intervals; 5 min rest in zone 2 2 hr **Alternate Workout:** Group ride—aggressive	**END** 3 hr
Total hours: 10:30:00							
4	Rest day	Rest day	**END** with 1 × [5 × 1 min in zone 6; 2 min rest]. Rest 5–8 min between sets 1 hr	IF RACING SATURDAY: **Rest day** IF RACING SUNDAY: **END** with 1 × [5 × 1 min in zone 6; 2 min zone 1]. Rest 5 min between sets 1 hr	IF RACING SATURDAY: **Prerace short:** **END** with 3 × 90 sec [zone 5]; 5 min rest 30 min IF RACING SUNDAY: **Rest day**	IF RACING SUNDAY: **Prerace short:** **END** with 3 × 90 sec [zone 5]; 5 min rest 30 min **OR** **Race!**	**Race!**
Bike hours: 2:00:00; Race hours: 4:00:00 Total hours: 6:00:00							

Abbreviations: END, endurance, zone 2; max VO$_2$, maximum VO$_2$, zone 5; SST, sweet spot, zone 3; tempo, zone 3.

Time Trial

One rider against the clock, the race of truth, *contre-la-montre*—whatever you call them, time trials are the races that define the best of the best in cycling. Riders start off one at a time and compete against the clock to post the fastest time on courses ranging from a few kilometers to over 60 kilometers in length. There is no drafting allowed, so riders' times are defined by their ability, pacing, and mental strength. Winning a time trial requires the ability to stay focused despite all the pain in your body, the variations of the course, or concerns over your competitors. You must learn to ignore the voice that tells you to slow down, stop, you can't do this—you must keep pedaling as fluidly, quickly, and powerfully as possible.

Races against the clock aren't limited to licensed road competitions or triathlons—even the most casual among us can find ourselves pegged at our power threshold in a desperate bid to get to the grocery store before it closes or finish our commute in time to clean up before the morning meeting. When you find yourself counting seconds, here are some strategies you can use to achieve at least a temporary victory over time itself.

RIDE AT YOUR THRESHOLD

In the past few years, the point at which you can sustain a high level of power for an extended period of time has been associated with several terms, such as anaerobic threshold, lactic threshold, and power threshold. All of them get to the same idea: You want to find the magic point that lets you ride as hard as you can for as long as you need to. Go too fast and you blow up and must ease off to recover; pedal too slowly and you finish with energy you should have used. You don't need a power meter or heart rate monitor to find this zone: just ride hard enough so that when you try to speak, you can get out only a few words at a time rather than complete sentences or even long phrases. That's your optimal extended time trial speed.

GET AERO

Most people think of equipment—aero bars, deep-dish rims, skinsuits—when they imagine ways to cheat the wind. A lot of speed is free: When you're in a hurry, scoot your butt back on the saddle and ride with your hands in the drops. (If you have a flat bar, scooting back and bending your elbows will still lower your profile, making you more aerodynamic.) On descents, tuck your elbows and knees in toward your bike and lower your head as much as possible while still maintaining control. If you need just one bottle, put it in the cage on your seat tube, where it's slightly more aero, instead of on your down tube. If you're riding in street shoes, tuck your laces into your shoes instead of letting them flap—every millisecond counts, right?

STAY SMOOTH

In a group—say when you're barreling toward home to beat a storm—stay as close to others as you can while maintaining a steady pace. Smoothness trumps speed: If one rider in the group is uncomfortable riding as closely as everyone else wants to, that rider will likely form gaps or make the pace herky-jerky by braking and accelerating. Though it may seem frustrating, it's best to establish a uniform spacing the entire group can maintain. When you get to the front of a paceline, don't accelerate dramatically or sprint past the receding rider. Instead, maintain the group's speed. If you feel strong and want to increase the pace, do so gradually over the course of your turn. Big jumps in pace break up the group and harm your overall average speed.

Pro Tip

Be extra cautious during the first 10 minutes of a rainstorm, when oil and dust float to the pavement's surface but haven't yet washed away. However, painted road lines and steel surfaces (manhole covers, grates, railroad tracks, bridge decks, and expansion joints) get slippery right away and stay treacherous until they are completely dry.

DIY AERO

On a flat road, as much as 95 percent of a rider's energy is used to overcome wind resistance, says Todd Carver, who runs Retül, a bike-fitting company in Boulder, Colorado. Just 20 percent of that drag comes from the bike—the other 80 percent is from you. By tweaking your road bike for fit and efficiency, you can smooth the air flow around your bike and body. Here's how.

1. **ATTACH CLIP-ON AERO BARS.** Don't worry about the position at this point—you'll tweak it later.

2. **MOVE THE SADDLE FORWARD AND/OR SWAP YOUR SEATPOST**. One of the most common conversion fit mistakes is slapping on aero bars but leaving the saddle where it is. If you're effectively moving the handlebar forward, you need to move your body too. Think of it as rotating yourself forward around the bottom bracket, like hands on a clock. Your elbows should be 2 to 3 cm behind the rear edge of the aero bar pads, with a roughly 110-degree angle at the elbow. For road bike fit, a plumb line dropped from the rider's forward knee (with crankarms level) should pass just in front of the pedal spindle. For ideal tri fit, you want your knee farther forward, 1 additional centimeter in front of the pedal spindle for every centimeter of

height difference between the saddle and the aero bar pads. You may need a two-position post, depending on how much adjustment your seat rails offer.

3. **CORRECT SADDLE HEIGHT AND ANGLE.** Moving a seat forward also effectively lowers it. You want about a 30-degree bend in your knee when the crankarms are perpendicular to the ground. (Note: This is a different measure than the one used for road bike fit.) A normal road position has a level seat, but for a multisport fit, you should rotate the saddle downward 1 degree for every centimeter of drop between the seat and the aero bar pads, up to 8 degrees. This will allow you to roll your hips forward and open up your hip angle for a more natural pedaling style. Make these adjustments at the same time as Step 2, as one measurement affects the other.

4. **DIAL IN YOUR BACK ANGLE.** If the aero extensions are too high, move a steerer-tube spacer or two above the stem, or flip a positive-angle stem upside down, or both. Ideally, your back will be flat like Dave Zabriskie's, but spinal flexibility may limit you. If the bars are too low, consider a higher rise stem.

5. **TWEAK YOUR BARS.** The key here is to decrease frontal area as much as comfortably possible. Align the elbow pads so your elbows sit directly in line with your hands.

It's fine to create a wider "stance" on the bar by increasing the distance between the extensions; just keep your forearms pointing straight, not angled inward, which increases drag.

If, after some break-in time, you can't stay in your tuck over the distance of your goal race (cornering, climbing, and tricky descents excluded), then your position is too aggressive, says Scott Holz, bike-fit expert and global manager of Specialized Bicycle Component University. For sprint tris or time trials that last less than an hour, your position should be as aggressive as you can tolerate. For Olympic-distance events or a 40-K time trial, increase your torso angle 5 degrees. For a half-Ironman, add 5 to 10 degrees, and for a full Ironman, 10 or more degrees.

When in doubt, choose comfort over aerodynamics. You'll go faster in a less aerodynamic position if you can reliably produce lots of power over a longer period of time. That said, with any aero position you will probably give up some amount of power compared with your road position, but that's okay. "Cyclists are macho and like to focus on power," says University of Utah researcher Jim Martin, PhD, who consults on aerodynamic efficiency with the Australian Institute of Sport. "If you give up a few percentage points in power output, but gain that same amount in aerodynamic efficiency, you'll still go faster."

TRAINING PLAN

This plan is for the road cyclist who wants to do a time trial race and has between 7 and 12 hours a week to train. To ensure you are ready to complete this plan, you should have already completed 4 to 6 weeks of "base" training totaling at least 500 miles of riding. The plan consists of workouts at various effort levels. It offers wattage, heart rate, and rate of perceived exertion options so you can gauge your effort whether you use a power meter, a heart rate monitor, or prefer to work out by feel.

Workouts

BURSTS: Ride in zone 2. Vary cadence throughout the ride and work on your pedaling form. Practice "coming over the top" and "pulling through the bottom" of the pedal (pretend there is glass in your shoes). Cadence: 85 to 105.

START INTERVALS: Start with one foot on the ground in a 53 × 16 gear (approximately). Practice clipping in and building up to 500+ watts. Rest for 3 to 4 minutes in between.

SST INTERVALS: Complete 2 x 12-minute intervals in the "Sweet Spot" (zone 3.5) with 5 minutes recovery in between. Ride all other time in level 2 endurance zone. Note: The sweet spot is a small area of intensity characterized by 88 to 93 percent of one's functional threshold power.

Ready for Your Next Challenge?

Download our hill climb training plan at Bicycling.com/hillclimbtraining.

Time Trial Training Plan

WEEK	MONDAY	TUESDAY	WEDNESDAY	THURSDAY	
1	Rest day	**END** with 3 × 10 min (zone 4); 5 min rest 1 hr, 15 min on time trial bike	**END** 1 hr, 30 min	Eight Start Intervals + 10 min active recovery/light **END** with 4 × 6 min (zone 5); 6 min rest 1 hr, 15 min on time trial bike Note: Cadence should be one gear harder then you typically pedal, with a target cadence of 75–85. (If you are hitting power targets, go for a fifth interval!!)	

Total hours: 9:30:00

2	Rest day	**END** with 4 × 10 min (zone 4); 5 min rest 1 hr, 30 min on time trial bike	**END** 2 hr on road bike	**END** with 3 × 15 min (zone 4); 5 min rest 1 hr, 30 min on time trial bike	

Total hours: 10:30:00

3	Rest day	**END** with 6 × 2 min (zone 6); 4 min rest 1 hr, 30 min on time trial bike Note: Using a big gear, really accelerate during the last 15 seconds of the interval.	**END** with 30 min zone 3 1 hr, 30 min 2 hr	Eight Start Intervals + 10 min active recovery/light **END** with 5 × 6 min (zone 5); 6 min rest 1 hr, 30 min on time trial bike Note: Cadence should be "one gear" harder then you typically pedal with a target cadence of 75–85. (If you are hitting power targets, go for a fifth interval!!)	

Total hours: 11:30:00

4	Rest day	Rest day	**END** with 3 × 2 min (zone 6); 4 min rest 1 hr on time trial bike Note: Using a big gear, really accelerate during the last 15 seconds of each interval.	IF RACING SATURDAY: **Rest day** IF RACING SUNDAY: **END** 3 × 3 min (zone 5); 3 min rest 1 hr, 30 min on time trial bike	

Total hours: 5:30:00
Bike hours: 1:30:00; Race hours: 4:00:00

Abbreviations: END, endurance/zone 2; tempo, zone 3.

FRIDAY	SATURDAY	SUNDAY
Active recovery 1 hr on time trial bike	**END** with 2 × 12 min (zone 3.5); 5 min rest 2 hr, 15 min on the time trial bike	**END with Bursts** 2 hr, 15 min on road bike
Active recovery 1 hr on time trial bike Note: You get faster when you are resting and recovering, not when you are working hard!! Rest days are about going easy enough to really allow your legs to recover, so no hard efforts, take it easy, and look at the scenery.	**END** with 6 × 2 min (zone 6); 4 min rest 2 hr on time trial bike Note: Using a big gear, really accelerate during the last 15 seconds of the interval. If you want, you can ride for an hour at endurance pace BEFORE this and then a hour after to make it a long ride on your time trial bike. Get used to the position.	**END** with 2 × 12 min (zone 3.5); 5 min recovery 2 hr, 30 min
Active recovery 1 hr on time trial bike	**SST Intervals** 2 hr, 30 min on time trial bike	**END** with Bursts 3 hr on time trial or road bike
IF RACING SATURDAY: **END** with 3 × 90 sec (zone 5); 5 min rest 30 min IF RACING SUNDAY: **Rest day**	IF RACING SUNDAY: **END** with 3 × 90 sec (zone 5); 5 min rest 30 min **Or Race!**	**Race!**

CHAPTER 12

Cyclocross

I like cyclocross because it's a spastic scurry just like my life.

—LISA MUHICH, MULTI-TIME NATIONAL CYCLOCROSS CHAMPION

FALL IS A GREAT TIME OF YEAR FOR CYCLISTS. YOUR FITNESS IS at its peak after a summer of riding, the weather is cooling off, and changing leaves make for scenic views. Best of all, it's the beginning of cyclocross season.

Cyclocross was developed in the early 1900s, primarily in Europe, as a way for road racers to squeeze in off-season training, and events still traditionally take place in the fall and winter. It's now the fastest-growing two-wheeled discipline in the United States, and many riders are making it their primary discipline.

How It Works

Riders complete multiple laps on timed, closed, off-road courses of 1 to 3 miles that include obstacles such as wooden barriers, steep run-ups, and sand pits that require riders to dismount and carry their bikes. Most amateur events take 40 to 45 minutes to finish. Riders wear mountain bike shoes with grippy treads but ride cyclocross-specific bikes.

The Appeal

"There's something for everyone in 'cross," says six-time national champion Tim Johnson, who rides for the Cannondale/Cyclocrossworld.com team. Riders below the elite level have discovered that cyclocross is less intimidating and time-consuming than other disciplines. You don't have to think about traffic; there's no road rash, no 40-plus mph descents, no strict code of conduct or overwhelming snobbishness about gear or apparel. "In 'cross, no one gives a rat's ass what you wear," says Brad Ross, who runs Cross Crusade, an Oregon-based cyclocross series. And because you're doing laps, you don't have to worry about being dropped.

What to Expect

Rowdy, possibly inebriated but well-intentioned spectators cheering from the sidelines. Races are often staged in city parks near playgrounds, picnic tables, and barbecues. Ross, who also designs courses, often plots out a cloverleaf pattern, which means riders are constantly in view. "As a spectator, you can see the whole race by standing in one place," he says. "Preferably in the beer garden." Many cyclocross races have a festival-like vibe: People pitch tents, play music, and trade war stories around campfires. "It creates a bond that's closer than any sport I've ever done," says Tim Rutledge, marketing manager for Seattle's Redline Bicycles and former US cyclocross champion.

Pro Tip

At a race, take a few practice laps during your warm-up to develop a strategy for how to approach barriers and run-ups.

Get Your Bike Cyclocross Fit

Five ways to prep your ride for the muddy, gritty, and not-so-pretty cyclocross season.

START FRESH

Replace cables and housing at your tune-up, even if you don't think it's necessary. Dirt works its way inside housing lines, making shifting and braking gritty and slow. If you ride in sloppy conditions, ask your shop if it's possible to fully enclose cables in one uninterrupted length of housing.

RESPECT YOUR RIMS

After every race and wet ride, or every 100 miles, clean your rims. For caked-on crud, scrub with soapy water and rinse using a light shower setting. To remove grimy buildup, wipe with a dry rag and rubbing alcohol. If the ride was exceptionally wet, remove wheels and buff brake pad surfaces with an emery cloth.

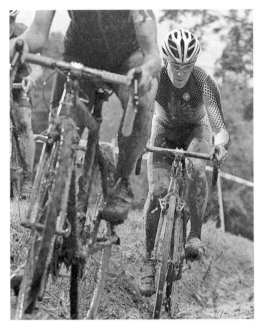
Muddy conditions help develop good bike-handling skills.

TREAD LIGHTLY

A general inflation rule: With one thumb across the rear tire and the palm of your other hand on top of it, push down with your body weight. If your thumb hits the rim, add air until it doesn't touch. For soft conditions, run your front tire 5 to 7 psi less than the rear. On hardpack, increase both tires by 5 to 10 psi.

PICK THE RIGHT TAPE

How much elbow grease you'll need to clean your bar tape depends on whether you prefer comfort or convenience. Padded tape reduces vibration but stains easily. Tacky tape gets dingy and is less padded, but it's grippy when wet and cleans up better. Leather tape is pricey but looks sharp and is easy to clean.

LUBE WHAT MOVES

In addition to your chain, which you should lubricate after every dusty or muddy ride, place a drop of oil on each pivot point on both derailleurs and the contact point between the brake arms and spring (if they're squeaking or not releasing from the rim). Always apply lube on a clean bike and wipe off the excess.

Skills

If you want to have fun while building fitness, it's tough to beat spending the autumn knee-deep in the mud of your local cyclocross scene. Before you compete, try to master a few essential techniques. "There's nothing more discouraging than losing time because you can't comfortably get off and back onto the saddle," says Adam Myerson, a professional road and cyclocross racer and the owner of Cycle-Smart Coaching. The key to speedy transitions, he says, is conserving your forward momentum. Here's how to do it.

OBSTACLES

ON YOUR LEFT. Enter the transition (any section that requires you to dismount) in the gear you want to exit in. Dismount on the left side of your bike to protect your legs

(continued on page 182)

THE CRUCIBLE

BY ADAM MYERSON, A PROFESSIONAL CYCLOCROSS RACER

IT'S NEARLY IMPOSSIBLE TO EXPLAIN CYCLOCROSS TO someone who has never seen it. "You do what with the bike? What if it rains? Do they ever cancel? You race in the SNOW?!" As a cyclocross rider, you find yourself at a loss trying to give people a sense of the difficulty, the absurdity, the degree of seriousness participants bring to the sport. In Portland, Oregon, every race is a hipster tractor pull where a thousand people will come out to play in incessant winter rain and mud. On the other side of the country there's Boston, with its manicured courses, expensive coaches, and compulsive race series points tracking, which is laughably puritanical but perhaps more pure.

Somewhere between these two extremes, somewhere in the middle on the Kinsey scale of love of mud, is the place where cyclocross racing is just raw, unadorned beauty. The effort feels like a 40-kilometer time trial in its intensity, like a 1-hour criterium in its relentless speed changes and dynamism. Sprint, brake, slide, turn, sprint as hard as you can, over and over. The demands of technique distract you from some of the physical pain. Sometimes you can forget how badly you're suffering if you have to back off the pedals for a second and try to negotiate an off-camber U-turn, with one foot out of the pedals like you're 6 years old again and bombing the turn into your driveway on your BMX bike. You pause, take a deep breath, rip your bike like a slot car around a plastic stake marking the edge of the course, and try not to laugh out loud while doing it. Or maybe, just let yourself laugh.

Sometimes, though, cyclocross really is just unrelentingly and completely hard. Voluntarily getting out of your car when it's 33 degrees and raining, and you are wearing nothing but a spandex jumpsuit, is sometimes a better story after the fact than it is a worthwhile experience while it's happening. Your car is never far away, you can quit at any time, and still you plod along, shoes full of ice water. Soon you can't feel your hands, which means you can't shift or steer, and you crash in a turn while the rider you were hanging on to like a piece of flotsam in a cold, dead ocean pedals away. You stand yourself up. You clean mud out of your teeth. You know you are done, that you will never do anything this ridiculous again.

Then the race ends. The feeling in your hands comes back, more painful than when they froze initially. Eventually you get home, take a warm shower, begin to put distance between you and the misery. Over the next few days, the memory of the pain fades and you're left with thoughts of how you could have taken a better line through that one turn. How amazing it was to dismount your bike at 20 miles an hour with a punk-rock marching band putting up a wall of sound around you on the other side of the course tape. You thought you were going to die at the time, but now all you can think of is how much fun you had, how you'd do it again if you could, how you'd do it differently next time. You're left, finally, with the feeling of joy and satisfaction that comes with self-inflicted torment—the essence of endurance sports.

With cyclocross, you can have that manic cycle every week if you want. Every Saturday or Sunday—or both—there's another race, with more joy, more pain, more passion, more satisfaction, and another opportunity to create an amazing story to tell—a story about something you never want to experience while it's happening but that leaves you with a feeling you long for once the anguish is passed. That is what cyclocross is all about. It's like real life, but better.

from your drivetrain. As you coast toward the barrier, unclip your left foot and shift your weight onto your left instep. When you're ready to dismount, unclip and swing your right leg around the back of the bike and move your right hand to the top tube about 6 inches in front of the seatpost. Coasting with your right foot behind the left, hit the ground with your right. Begin running with the left.

CARRY THE WEIGHT. It's easier and faster to shoulder your bike for uphill runs, stairs, and muddy sections. As you dismount, instead of grabbing the top tube, reach through the frame and grasp the down tube near the bottle cage area. Lift the front of the top tube onto your right shoulder. Then wrap your right arm around the down tube and grab the left drop

of your handlebar with your right hand to hold the bike securely.

BIKE BARRIERS. Don't lift your bike so that your saddle goes into your armpit; you may hit the barrier or trip over your pedals. Instead, place your right hand palm-down on the top tube and take Myerson's advice: "Keep your elbow between you and your bike," he says. "This helps to move the bike a little farther away from your body so you can lift it to shoulder height."

REMOUNT. "You want to run onto your bike the way a track hurdler steps over a hurdle," Myerson says. "This keeps your momentum moving forward." The remount starts with both hands on the tops or hoods of the handlebar. Running on the left side of the bike, look forward and keep your hips in the area

EVOLVED SPECIES

HOW ARE CYCLOCROSS BIKES DIFFERENT FROM ROAD bikes? Let us count the ways.

1. The tires are wider and slightly knobbier in order to grip wet, mucky slopes.
2. A wide-angle centerpull cantilever brake offers better mud clearance.
3. The top tube is sometimes flat underneath for better comfort and stability when perched on a shoulder.
4. To accommodate wider tires, the rear end is often longer by an average of 10 to 15 mm. The longer wheelbase also adds stability when you're powering around sloppy corners.
5. For additional stability, head angles are often lower by a degree and bottom brackets are lower, too (relative to the axle height).

CAN I USE A MOUNTAIN BIKE IN A CYCLOCROSS RACE?

IT'S NOT UNCOMMON FOR FIRST-TIMERS TO SHOW up at a cyclocross race with a mountain bike. "I started racing on one," says Jeremy Powers, a pro cyclocross rider for Aspire Racing. A flat handlebar and a suspension fork might earn you a little extra heckling, but don't let that stop you from partaking in the fun, if the rules allow it. Most local races permit mountain bikes as long as the handlebar doesn't have bar ends. Races sanctioned by the Union Cycliste Interationale (professional cycling's international governing body), however, prohibit bikes with flat handlebars. "A mountain bike is also heavier," Powers says. If you're not up for buying a dedicated cyclocross bike, consider swapping out the mountain bike tires, which add weight and don't roll as fast over grass.

between the cranks and saddle. Push off your left foot, open your hips to the right, and drive your right knee forward over the saddle. "Like the trailing leg of a hurdler, catch the saddle with the inside of your right thigh," Myerson says. Then bring your right foot down onto the pedal. Twist your hips closed and feather the inner thigh of your mounting leg onto the saddle, then square your hips to the bar as you slide into place. Aim for a glide, not a plop.

ON THE DESCENT

LET IT ROLL. When the going gets steep and muddy, cyclocross pro Gina Hall focuses on letting her bike roll. "If you hit your brakes, you're more likely to slide out," she explains. For a scary-steep descent, stand up, get your

weight back over the rear wheel, keep your hands in the drops (so you can be ready to brake, just in case), and stay loose. "Mostly, it's mental. Your bike can roll through pretty much anything. It's your mind that will make you crash." Of course, even Hall admits that some trails deserve caution: "If

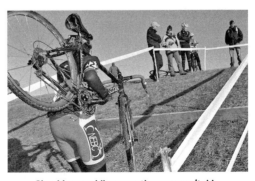

Shoulder your bike on sections you can't ride.

it's really slippery, I'll take one foot out of the pedal and use it for balance to ward off a fall," she says.

THROUGH SHARP TURNS

STAY CENTERED. Successfully slinging your bike through a slick hairpin turn is largely a matter of weight distribution. "Keep your body positioned over the center of the bike, even when you're leaning the bike into a turn," Hall says. By keeping your weight evenly distributed, you're less likely to have a wheel lose traction and slide out. "To stay centered, keep most of your body weight on the outside pedal, even if you're pedaling through the corner," Hall says. This helps your tires grip the ground, so you can hammer through the turn.

DO THE BUNNY HOP

At races, people line up by the jumps to see the riders bunny hop. Just learning the motion—even if you can't quite do it—will translate into being smoother and more in control over obstacles.

To learn to bunny hop, put a barrier in your yard—two boards nailed together at a right angle, so if you hit it, it falls. Try one 4 inches high or less to start. Lower your seat at least 4 inches to practice; raise it as you get better.

Try the whole hop motion at once. Lean back and pull your front wheel off the ground. To lift up the rear, think about pushing the bike forward. That will suck the rear wheel up

without feeling like you're pulling up with your legs. Remember to bend your arms and legs to land smoothly.

Pro Tip

Descending with someone who can do it better than you is a great way to learn and gain more confidence. If you see others pedal through a turn, you know you can pedal through. And though it's easy for someone else to say "relax," it really is true—if you tighten up and don't think you can do it, you're in for a pretty painful descent.

Training Plan

Racing cyclocross is a blast. You get to be a kid again, ride your bike over stuff, splash through puddles, get stuck in mud bogs, and of course have some fun racing with your friends. It is fast and intense and you will have to push your limits to beat the competition.

This plan is built for the beginner cyclocross racer who has a basic level of fitness from cycling and 6 to 8 hours to train weekly. (Ready for an intermediate or advanced plan? Check out bicycling.com/cyclocrosstraining.) You'll notice each weekend has 3 options: Plan A, Plan B, Plan C. Please select one of them to follow weekly. Here is the breakdown:

PLAN A is the plan to follow if you are racing on that Saturday.

PLAN B is the plan to follow if you are racing on that Sunday.

PLAN C is the plan to follow if you are NOT racing at all on the weekend.

WORKOUTS

30/30/30/30: On your local course or a course created at your local school or park, complete the following; 2 × 10 minutes (30-30-30-30, which is 30 seconds riding hard as you can, 30 seconds not pedaling and coasting, 30 seconds dismount and running fast, 30 seconds not pedaling and coasting. Repeat.) Ride 10 minutes easy. Then complete 4 minutes (zone 6) × 2 minutes (zone 1). Ride 10 minutes easy. Finish with 10 × 1 minute fast pedaling (1 minute on, 1 minute off). Cadence goal: 110 rpm.

ANAEROBIC CAPACITY POWER BUILDERS: Ride to a grass course featuring a hill with a 5 to 8 percent grade (the hill can be part of the course) then do 8 × 90-second hill climb intervals at maximum effort. Complete the first 75 seconds of each interval seated, then stand and power the last 15 seconds. Recover for 3 minutes in between intervals.

BIKE LIFTS: Complete 2 × 20 bike lifts before starting the cycling workout. The process is simple: Grab your top tube and lift the bike overhead. Put your water bottle on first to add a little weight.

BRICK: Immediately following the bike workout, run at a steady pace for a prescribed time. This should be done on grass and in cyclocross shoes or sneakers.

BURSTS: Sprint for 15 to 25 seconds at 200 percent of functional threshold power. Pick a variety of terrains: short climbs, long flats, downhill.

HILL SPRINTS: Find a steep grass-covered hill of 20 to 30 meters, hopefully part of your local training course. Immediately following the main set of your bicycle workout, completed five sprint intervals uphill, carrying the bike. Practice getting your knees high and find a good balance with the bike.

LACTATE THRESHOLD INTERVALS WITH BURSTS: Complete 3 × 10-minute intervals in zone 3 or 4. During each interval put in five "burst sprints" of 10 to 15 seconds at 150 percent of interval effort. Rest 5 to 8 minutes between each set.

MICRO BURSTS: Using a your local cross-training course, complete 3 × 10-minute "microburst" intervals with 5 minutes rest in between sets. A burst is 15 seconds ON (zone 6) and 15 seconds OFF (zone 1). Repeat continually for 10 minutes.

SWEET SPOT (SST) CRISSCROSS INTERVALS: On the grass, complete 2 × 10-minute intervals at zone 3 or 4, then every 2 minutes pop it up to zone 6 for 30 seconds, recover back to zone 3 or 4, but nothing lower! Rest 5 to 8 minutes between sets.

Cyclocross Training Plan

WEEK	MONDAY	TUESDAY	WEDNESDAY	THURSDAY	FRIDAY	SATURDAY	SUNDAY
1	Rest day	**Bike:** END with 7 Bursts 1 hr, 30 min **Run:** Brick 20 min	**Strength:** Bike lifts 15 min **Bike:** 1hr END with 30 min Tempo 1 hr, 30 min	**Bike:** END with 7 Bursts 1 hr, 30 min **Run:** Brick 30 min	**Plan A:** **Bike:** END with 3 × 90 sec max VO_2 intervals; 5 min rest 1 hr, 30 min **Plans B and C:** **Bike:** Active recovery 1 hr	**Plan A:** Race **Plan B:** **Bike:** END with 3 × 90 sec max VO_2 intervals; 5 min rest 1 hr, 30 min **Plan C:** **Bike:** 10-min Micro bursts 1 hr, 30 min	**Plans A and C:** **Bike:** END 2 hr, 30 min **Plan B:** Race
2	Rest day	**Bike:** END with 2 × 10-min SST Crisscross intervals + 10 min Active Recovery + 2 × 5 max VO_2 intervals; 3 min rest 1 hr, 22 min **Run:** Brick 30 min	**Strength:** Bike lifts 15 min **Bike:** 1hr END with 30 min Tempo 1 hr, 30 min	**Bike:** END with 2 × 10-min SST Crisscross intervals + 10 min Active Recovery + 2 × 5 max VO_2 intervals; 3 min rest 1 hr, 22 min	**Plan A:** **Bike:** END + 3 × 90 sec max VO_2 intervals; 5 min rest 1 hr, 30 min **Plans B and C:** **Bike:** Active recovery 1 hr	**Plan A:** Race **Plan B:** **Bike:** END with 3 × 90 sec. max VO_2 intervals; 5 min rest 1 hr, 30 min **Plan C:** **Bike:** 10-min Micro bursts 1 hr, 30 min	**Plans A and C:** **Bike:** END 2 hr, 30 min **Plan B:** Race
3	Rest day	**Bike:** END with 3 × 10-min lactate threshold intervals with bursts 1 hr, 21 min **Run:** Brick 30 min	**Strength:** Bike lifts 15 min **Bike:** 1hr END + 30 min Tempo 1 hr, 30 min	**Bike:** END with 3 × 10-min lactate threshold intervals with bursts 1 hr, 22 min	**Plan A:** **Bike:** END with 3 × 90 sec max VO_2 intervals; 5 min rest 1 hr, 30 min **Plans B and C:** **Bike:** Active recovery 1 hr	**Plan A:** Race **Plan B:** **Bike:** END with 3 × 90 sec max VO_2 intervals; 5 min rest 1 hr, 30 min **Plan C:** **Bike:** 10-min Micro bursts 1 hr, 30 min	**Plans A and C:** **Bike:** END 2 hr, 30 min **Plan B:** Race
4	Rest day	Rest day	**Bike:** END with 7 Bursts 1 hr, 15 min	**Bike:** Active recovery 1 hr	**Plan A:** **Bike:** END + 3 × 90 sec max VO_2 intervals; 5 min rest 1 hr, 30 min **Plans B and C:** **Bike:** Active recovery 1 hr	**Plan A:** Race **Plan B:** **Bike:** END with 3 × 90 sec max VO_2 intervals; 5 min rest 1 hr, 30 min **Plan C:** **Bike:** 10-min Micro bursts 1 hr, 30 min	**Plans A and C:** **Bike:** END 2 hr, 30 min **Plan B:** Race

Abbreviations: END, endurance/zone 2; max VO_2, maximum VO_2/zone 5; SST, tempo, zone 3.

WEEK	MONDAY	TUESDAY	WEDNESDAY	THURSDAY	FRIDAY	SATURDAY	SUNDAY
5	Rest day	**Bike:** 30/30/30/30 1 hr, 45 min **Run:** Hill sprints 30 min	**Strength:** Bike lifts 15 min **Bike:** END with 3 × 10-min Micro bursts intervals; 5 min rest 1 hr	**Bike:** END with 2 × 10-min SST Crisscross intervals + 10 min Active Recovery + 2 × 5 max VO_2 intervals; 3 min rest 1 hr, 22 min	**Plan A:** **Bike:** END with 3 × 90 sec max VO_2 intervals; 5 min rest 1 hr, 30 min **Plans B and C:** **Bike:** Active recovery 1 hr	**Plan A:** Race **Plan B:** **Bike:** END with 3 × 90 sec max VO_2 intervals; 5 min rest 1 hr, 30 min **Plan C:** **Bike:** 10-min Micro bursts 1 hr, 30 min	**Plans A and C:** **Bike:** END 2 hr, 30 min **Plan B:** Race
6	Rest day	**Bike:** 30/30/30/30 1 hr, 45 min **Strength:** Bike lifts 15 min	**Run:** Hill sprints 1 hr, 30 min **Bike:** AC Power Builders + 10 min END + 1 × 20 min in zone 3 or 4 1 hr, 30 min	**Bike:** Active recovery 1 hr	**Plan A:** **Bike:** END with 3 × 90 sec max VO_2 intervals; 5 min rest 1 hr, 30 min **Plans B and C:** **Bike:** Active recovery 1 hr	**Plan A:** Race **Plan B:** **Bike:** END with 3 × 90 sec. max VO_2 intervals; 5 min rest 1 hr, 30 min **Plan C:** **Bike:** 10-min Micro bursts 1 hr, 30 min	**Plans A and C:** **Bike:** END 2 hr, 30 min **Plan B:** **Race**
7	Rest day	**Bike:** 30/30/30/30 1 hr, 30 min **Strength:** Bike lifts 15 min	**Run:** Hill sprints 30 min **Bike:** END with 10-min Micro bursts 1 hr, 30 min	Rest day	**Plan A:** **Bike:** END with 3 × 90 sec. max VO_2 intervals; 5 min rest 1 hr, 30 min **Plans B and C:** **Bike:** Active recovery 1 hr	**Plan A:** Race **Plan B:** **Bike:** END with 3 × 90 sec. max VO_2 intervals; 5 min rest 1 hr, 30 min **Plan C:** **Bike:** 10-min Micro bursts 1 hr, 30 min	**Plans A and C:** **Bike:** END 2 hr, 30 min **Plan B:** Race
8	Rest day	**Bike:** Active recovery 1 hr **Run:** Brick 30 min	**Bike:** 30/30/30/30 1 hr, 30 min **Strength:** Bike lifts 15 min	Rest day	**Plan A:** **Bike:** END with 3 × 90 sec. max VO_2 intervals; 5 min rest 1 hr, 30 min **Plans B and C:** **Bike:** Active recovery 1 hr	**Plan A:** Race **Plan B:** **Bike:** END with 3 × 90 sec max VO_2 intervals; 5 min rest 1 hr, 30 min **Plan C:** **Bike:** 10-min Micro bursts 1 hr, 30 min	**Plans A and C:** **Bike:** END 2 hr, 30 min **Plan B:** Race

CHAPTER 13

Mountain Biking

A mountain bike race is a constant hard effort for two or three hours. In road racing the efforts often come in surges. You ride easy for a while then you have to make an extreme, hard effort. They are two different efforts, two different forms of suffering.

—John Tomac, US former cross-country and downhill mountain bike champion, cross-country world champion, and World Cup champion

IN 2013 I GOT AN EMAIL FROM WORLD CHAMPION MOUNTAIN biker Rebecca Rusch (aka the Queen of Pain) inviting me out to Sun Valley, Idaho, for a week to participate in her SRAM Gold Rusch Tour, a series of events Rebecca runs to encourage more women to get on bikes. She also casually mentioned that USA Cycling's mountain bike marathon national championships would also take place in town at the end of the week and I was welcome to register. It had been years since I had been on a mountain bike (even then I only rode casually on fairly benign trails), but I thought, "what the heck" and signed up.

Needless to say, I found myself in a bit over my head. The hills were mountains and the trail edges were cliffs. I had never ridden such challenging—and frightening—terrain and spent the first 3 days of camp white-knuckling my handlebars and grabbing way too much brake. Lucky for me, Rebecca was an apt and patient teacher and not only did I complete her camp, but I finished the race, too—all 40 miles and 6,000+ feet of elevation gain. I was elated.

You don't have to be a mud stud to race a

mountain bike. As I learned, off-road races are one of the best ways to improve your skills, find new places to ride, and have a ton of fun. This expert-approved advice will get you started.

Eight Essential Skills

If you want to learn how to shred, who better to learn from than the masters? What follows are riding tips from coach Tom Hillard, who started Specialized technical support, and pros Wayne Croasdale, Ned Overend, Silvia Fürst, Jeff Osguthorpe, Peter Swenson, Golden Brainard, Todd Tanner, and Steve Tilford.

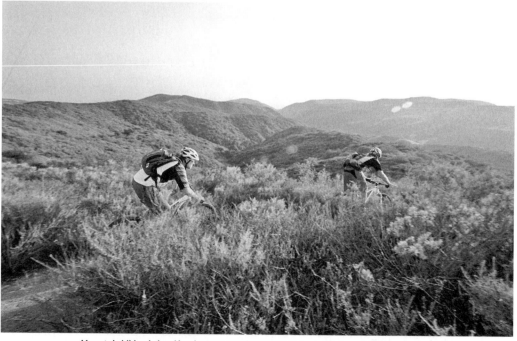

Mountain biking is hard but it can reward you with some pretty breathtaking scenery.

PASSING

What the Coach says:

"If you can pass someone on singletrack and the riders behind you can't get around, you can put a lot of distance on them quickly. Ideal passing situations are when the trail widens a bit or splits in two for a few feet. But to see this you've got to look past the rider in front of you. Find a spot or several corners near the finish and get them dialed perfectly. These are the places where you can make your move."

THE DRILL: "Get a partner and have him [or her] ride down singletrack at about 80 percent of maximum speed. Pass him, riding at 90 to 100 percent. Then slow to 80 percent and let him pass you. Keep leapfrogging this way."

What the Pros say:

TILFORD: "Sometimes you have to wait until later in a race when people are tired. Then, when you see about two handlebar widths' room, come on strong and tell them which side you're on. Also, the start is so important because if the course narrows to singletrack, you'll be stuck and can lose a lot of time. That's why it's important to train to get your heart rate up high for a short period, then back off to avoid blowing up."

FÜRST: "If possible, always pass on the inside of a turn because the distance is shorter."

CLIMBING

What the Coach says:

"Keep just enough weight on the front wheel to maintain steering ability. As the hill gets steeper, shift your weight forward by moving your upper body closer to the handlebar and sliding forward on the saddle. In rocky conditions you'll need to stand to allow the bike to float underneath you. This also gives you more power to heave up and over larger rocks and ledges, and more control over what the back wheel is doing."

THE DRILL: "For maximum traction, get to know where your back wheel is. A lot of riders don't know that the back and front tires follow different lines, with the rear going inside the path of the front. Place a rock on smooth ground and make repeated figure eights around it. First pass the front wheel to the outside of the rock and the rear to the inside, coming as close to it with the rear as possible. Then pass both wheels around the outside, again coming as close to the rock as possible. Finally, pass the front wheel around the outside of the rock and roll over it with the rear."

What the Pros say:

OVEREND: "The worst thing to do on a steep climb is to move your body weight forward as you would on a road bike. This takes your weight off the rear wheel, and you lose traction. Instead, bend at the waist and pull back on the bar, not up. Don't mash the pedals. Pedal in circles, so power pulses don't cause the wheel to break loose. You want your legs to be turning over fast enough to keep momentum over obstacles. One way to practice this is with one-legged pedaling. Drive your leg toward the bar, then drag your heel back. As you climb, think of what your neck and upper chest are doing. If these muscles are tense it will be hard to breathe. You don't want to use muscles that aren't required for the climb. I like to do a pronounced exhale once in a while, like Lamaze breathing, to relax."

CROASDALE: "For short climbs and rollers, use your momentum. Sprint into them, then downshift one click at a time as you come out. Really use those gears and try to pedal the whole thing."

SWENSON: "Keep a stable upper body. Once your head begins to rock, it can cause problems. You can get away with it on the road, but off-road excessive upper body movement can cause you to lose traction in the loose stuff. Also, you shouldn't have your hands on the bar ends if the trail is loose. That gives you too much turning torque, and the wheel will slide out."

SHIFTING

What the Coach says:

"Shifting is done as much with the eyes as it is with the hands. Most people don't anticipate.

For instance, if you wait until you're on the hill and can barely turn over the pedals, it's too late to downshift. In general, it's better to shift the front first because you can fine-tune the rear easier. Keep in mind that the new drivetrain systems are good, but you still have to back off pedal pressure somewhat."

THE DRILL: "Practice sitting and using the small chainring and standing while using the middle chainring on the same hill. See what works best for you. Keep in mind that if you can stand, once you crest the hill you can often accelerate away from other riders."

What the Pros say

FÜRST: "It's better to be in too small a gear and have to shift to a harder one. If the gear is too hard and you have to downshift, it's harder on the chain."

SWENSON: "Do a lot of little shifts to maintain cadence—even if it's just two teeth. And when you stand, go to one harder gear to maintain speed."

CORNERING

What the Coach says:

"Cornering can offer free speed if you do it right. There are three ways to position your body, as well as three lines you can take through a corner. That's a lot of combinations, but most people only know one. They tend instinctively to go into the corner way too soon and lean as if they're on a road bike. With this method you push your outside pedal down and countersteer by pushing the inside of the handlebar, 'carving' the turn. It's fast, but on a mountain bike you risk losing traction and sliding out.

"In many cases a better way is what I call the 'survival turn.' Your weight is to the inside, and your bike is upright. It's a good method if you don't know the corner, or if it's slippery and you need control. But it can be slower.

"Yet another method is for sand. Normally, if you keep your bike upright, you have to turn the handlebar more. But if you turn your bar in the sand, you'll wash out. Instead, turn it a minimal amount, leaning the bike underneath you while keeping your body upright. Use this any time you don't want your front wheel to dig in. Your line through a corner depends on where you make the apex [turning point]. A 'mid-apex' turn yields the highest average speed by creating a gentle arc and using every bit of the fire road. An 'early-apex' turn involves making the actual corner early, then powering out. The idea is to get the turn done and extend the straightaway coming out so you can go faster there. With a 'late-apex' turn you dive into the corner and do your actual turning later, extending the straightaway going into it. This means you can brake later and possibly pass someone going in. But you'll be slower coming out."

The drill: "Try using an early-, mid-, and late-apex turn in the same corner to see the advantages and disadvantages of each. Use cones to mark the turning point."

What the Pros say:

OSGUTHORPE: "I like the early-apex turn so I can get the corner done with. If you go for the late-apex, you'll almost always have to dump a lot of speed coming out."

CROASDALE: "The main thing is to come out of the corner fast. So I like to 'pre-turn' [early-apex]. This means I can come out fast, in a straight line."

FÜRST: "I like to put my weight to the inside and pedal through corners. It's like applying the gas in a car as you go around a curve—it helps maintain traction."

OBSTACLES

What the Coach says:

"So many riders coming from the road are stiff and don't move around on their bikes. Use your body weight to lunge up and over things. The first thing is to get your front wheel over. To do this you can simply yank on the handlebar, but that makes it hard to control how high the front end comes up. You can also pedal hard in a low gear. And with a suspension fork, you can push down and allow the rebound to raise the wheel. For most riders the best way is a combination, pushing on the pedals and pulling up on the bar at the same time. To get the back wheel over, pull the front wheel up as you abruptly push the bar forward. This causes the front end to drop and the back to rise. The other way is to pull up on the toe clips while in a standing position."

THE DRILL: "Place two pairs of cones a few feet apart. Elevate your front wheel when you pass through the first pair, and make it land at the second pair to practice controlling the amount of time the wheel is in the air. Or place a small rock or board on the ground, and elevate your front wheel just enough to graze it."

What the Pros say:

CROASDALE: "Everyone has a stronger leg—the same one you kick a ball with. Try to have that leg set up to apply pressure and get up and over an obstacle. Also, use a lot of upper-body motion. When your front wheel is midway over an obstacle, use your toe clips to lift the back wheel over. Your weight will be back, and then it will be thrown forward like a dolphin arcing through the water. You can also use one obstacle as a jump to get over the next one, such as when a 1-foot bump is followed by a small rock."

OVEREND: "Sometimes you need to use a 'stutter step' so your pedal doesn't hit a small obstacle. This means only taking the pedal halfway down, then lifting it back up to ensure clearance and pushing down again. Also, sometimes you need to surge just before the obstacle so you have the momentum to go over it. You don't want to be applying hard pedal pressure while you're on the obstacle because your rear wheel might break loose."

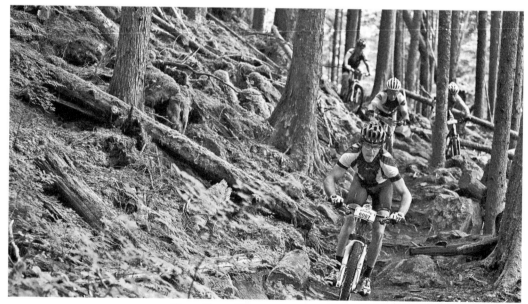

Move with your bike to maneuver obstacles.

TRAIL READING

What the Coach says:

"Looking ahead is critical in mountain biking. You must consider all your options in half a second, and a good rider will pick the right one. I call this 'sight reading,' and it's one reason John Tomac can fly down a trail he's never ridden before. He reads the trail better than the average rider. Look up the trail and see what's ahead. Is there a rut to avoid or a better line to take? Be constantly aware."

THE DRILL: "Practice looking up to a spot 20 to 30 meters ahead, and then down in front of your wheel. I'm convinced that the more you do this, the better you become at it. Pick a section and exaggerate this—be constantly scanning."

What the Pros say:

BRAINARD: "Sometime in training, stop your bike and read the terrain ahead. See what clues there are to help you ride that section. Is there a rut or some sand to avoid? Train your focus to switch back and forth, near and far. Think of it like looking up while you're driving, then down at your speedometer. Constantly go back and forth."

SWENSON: "People tend to just look at their front wheel, or the wheel ahead of them. They might know what's in the immediate corner, but not that it's followed by a short, steep ascent that requires a downshift. Look up the trail, and look through the bike ahead of you so you don't get stuck behind someone."

FÜRST: "Think of your eyes like a camera, taking a picture of what's ahead, then what's right in front. Record what you see."

BRAKING

What the Coach says:

"If you skid, you've failed. You need to find the maximum braking point, which is just before the tire starts skidding. It's better to slow gradually than lock up the brakes. Start by shifting your weight back, rising off the saddle, and extending your arms. As you get better, squeeze the front brake harder and the rear brake less, to prevent skidding. Motorcycle riders can brake so well that the rear wheel begins to leave the ground. Shoot for the point at which the rear tire still contacts the ground, but the braking is really happening in front."

THE DRILL: "Place some cones in the middle of a downhill that has a good runout. First apply the back brake only at that spot without skidding. Then apply both to see how much quicker you can stop. Then use just the front, being careful to avoid going over the bar.

"Another drill is to descend a steep hill as slowly as possible. Your tires will be on the verge of control and any mistake will cause you to fall, but you'll learn braking control. This can be hard. Some riders say the slower you go, the faster things happen."

What the Pros say:

OVEREND: "The front wheel can break loose in a turn if you brake too hard, so look for an area where you can get braking traction beforehand. Pull hard on both brakes when you're in the straightaway. But when you're in the turn, go easy on the front."

SWENSON: "The front brake is important, but lay off it in sand or loose stuff. You see people's forearms rippling trying to pull on the brakes in that kind of terrain. Instead, let the front wheel roll and carry a little more speed for a few seconds until you're through it."

TANNER: "Try to get comfortable when you're on the verge of locking up the wheels. Sometimes—if you can do it without ruining the trail—practice skidding with the rear wheel and letting go just before you slide out. This helps you get used to the feeling."

DESCENDING

What the Coach says:

"Keep your body in a neutral position, standing slightly off the saddle. This means that if you took your hands off the bar, you wouldn't fall forward or back. And remember that speed is your friend. Most of the time the faster you go, the more stable you are, due to the gyroscopic stability of the wheels. Also, falling is OK. What's not good is not knowing why you fell. Don't waste a perfectly good fall, or you'll just have to do it again. Treat it as a physics lesson."

The drill: "Mark a spot where you instinctively start braking for a downhill corner. The next time through, pick a spot that's farther forward. Keep moving this spot up until you find your personal maximum for the corner."

What the Pros say:

FÜRST: "Don't use straight arms on descents. People tend to tense and lock their arms when they should be using their arms and legs as suspension. Relax and try to be one with the bike. And if it's steep, move your weight back, behind the seat."

SWENSON: "Stay in touch with the saddle. Even if you're standing, pinch it with your thighs for control. Sometimes you can steer this way; you don't even need to turn the

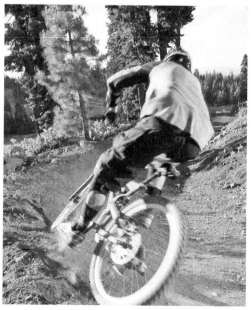

Stay off the brakes for more stability.

wheel. It helps you stay in control and know what the bike is doing."

TANNER: "Get set up early to change your line, before you get into trouble. Control your speed as you start. You've lost control if you have to skid in the middle."

TILFORD: "Don't be afraid to go straight down some rough sections and let your shock fork do the work. Sometimes that's the best way."

Rail a Berm

If you've ever been to a circus, you've probably seen the "cage of death," where a team of motorcycle riders zoom around the inside of a metal sphere just inches from a brave—and, of course, scantily clad—female assistant. Thanks to speed, the motorcycles stayed glued to the sides of the cage.

High-banked berms bring the same basic principle to mountain biking—though in most cases, without the assistant. If you have the right form and adequate speed, inertia will push your tires into the dirt so forcefully that the bike doesn't slide out, even when you lean way into the turn. With the perfect trail conditions that autumn brings, there's no better time to master berms. Here's how to get started.

LOOK, THEN LEAN

Study the berm's graceful arc before hitting it at speed. First, check the angle and height of the bank: The steeper it is, the more you can lean—your bike should be perpendicular to the bank—and the faster you can go. Next, find the grooved track where experienced riders have ridden the fastest line; that's the one you want to hit. Note how that line winds through the berm (a constant arc, low entrance/high exit, or high entrance/low exit) so you know where to go.

MOVE YOUR FINGERS

Enter the berm with your body in a ready position: standing on the pedals with cranks level, knees slightly bent; arms bent, elbows up and out, and eyes looking ahead. Force yourself to move your fingers off the brake levers and onto your bar, and keep them there until you exit.

LEAD WITH YOUR ELBOW

Don't stare at your front wheel or even at the apex of the turn—look ahead to the exit and you'll find it easier to stay on course. At the same time, be sure to keep your outside elbow (if it's a left turn, this is your right elbow) up and out. Focus on leading with that elbow as you lean into the berm. If the berm isn't as smooth as you thought, drop your outside pedal and put more weight into it to dig your tires in even more.

STEP ON THE GAS

Berms are all about speed. Go slowly and you'll be forced to the bottom of the berm, where you can't make use of the bank. Go faster, however, and your tires will drive into the more vertical surface as you lean in—you'll have phenomenal traction and gain speed because the berm will do the work of turning. On well-groomed, high-banked berms, you can ride ridiculously fast and still have an insane amount of traction.

PUMP IT UP

Once you get the hang of railing a berm with sheer speed, try pumping your bike through the turn to go even faster. As you approach the apex, lean forward and get lower on the bike. As you go through the apex, push the bar down and into your palms and extend your legs slightly. You'll move back on the bike somewhat as it scoots ahead to the exit. Zoom!

Do the Dreaded V-Dip

You're riding an epic loop that you've never done before. The singletrack is technical, but you're handling it well, and your pals behind are amazed at your stamina and prowess. Ahead you see the trail momentarily drop out of sight, only to reappear again just as fast. "Oh no," you say, "the Evil Dip!" (I'm not talking about an intellectually challenged serial killer, but rather the rhythm-killing, V-shaped trench found on trail rides.)

This particular dip drops a foot and a half, is 3 feet across, and has abrupt sides. Rather than dismount (getting dissed by your friends can be worse than a face-plant), you blaze ahead and try to clear the dip. But as the front wheel drops, you freeze up, grab a handful of front brake,

HOW TO PASS ON SINGLETRACK

Q: How should I let another mountain biker know I want to pass on the trail? And who has the right-of-way when you're going in opposite directions?

A: Good trail etiquette is not just a matter of safety; it's also about building community and making riders of all abilities feel welcome. So the most important thing is to be friendly. Instead of shouting that you're about to pass from behind, try saying something like, "Mind if I sneak by?" When you meet head-on, the rider going downhill should yield because it's harder to stop and restart when you're pedaling uphill. Regardless, resist the urge to get self-righteous about the rules. "If you make eye contact and smile you'll generally find that the pass goes smoothly," says Mark Eller of the International Mountain Bicycling Association. Also, remember that mountain bikers aren't the only trail users: Always yield to hikers and equestrians.

stuff the front wheel, fly over the bar, and pile-drive the opposite bank. Your nemesis approaches, pulls a little wheelie just as the front wheel is about to drop in, skims over the abyss and touches down lightly on the other side.

Abrupt dips, usually caused by swift runoff during rains, are common on most trails. Because they come in all shapes, sizes, and difficulties, the most valuable riding skill is reading the terrain to help you decide what to do. The severity of the dip, combined with your skill level, determines how you tackle it. There are typically four methods. I'll talk about three. The fourth is simply doing an Apollo 13 over the whole darn thing. If you can do that, heck, you don't need to read this section.

THE CYCLOCROSS CARRY

This technique is belittled for its lack of flare, but it's the right choice if the dip is particularly deep or, paradoxically, if you want to surmount the dip and proceed at maximum speed. Dismount just before the drop by slowing to a walking pace, unclipping the right foot, swinging it back over the rear wheel, then bringing it between the left foot and frame. Step forward onto the ground with the right foot while simultaneously releasing your left foot. This way you'll hit the ground running. Keep your left hand on the handlebar in its normal position; with your right, grasp the top tube and lift the bike like a suitcase, high enough to clear the ground as you jump across the dip. (We laid it out in steps, but in practice

it's one smooth motion.) Put the bike on the ground smoothly and grasp the bar with both hands, still moving forward. Now comes the tricky part: Throw your right leg up and over the back wheel and jump onto the saddle. Careful, though—don't land on your naughty bits, Lone Ranger–style. Instead, contact the saddle first with the inside of your right thigh, then slide into position.

THE ROLL-THROUGH

This one is flashier but with high carnage possibilities. Use it only for dips with rounded edges. If there's anything abrupt that might stop your wheel, try one of the other techniques. As you drop in, shift your weight to the rear; that's crucial. Then use your forward momentum, plus one or two well-timed pedal strokes and a judicious pull on the handlebar, to rocket your way out and forward. The flip side? (Ha-ha.) If your weight is too far forward upon entering the dip, your front wheel will stop dead, sending you over the bar. Practice and judgment are the keys to success. *Caution:* Be very careful with your front brake. In fact, make it a habit to enter dips without even touching your brake levers. The slightest squeeze can freeze the front wheel when otherwise it might have rolled through.

THE WHEELIE

This is the most advanced technique but also the one that, once mastered, is the most satisfying and useful for advanced trail riding. It's impressive as all get-out, too. At the lip of the drop, wheelie out into space: Shift your weight slightly to the rear, then simultaneously pull up on the bar while jamming hard on the pedals for one stroke. If your timing is good, the front wheel will land on the other side as the rear wheel drops into the dip. Momentum will (hopefully) allow you simply to roll up and out. Your forward motion may well stop you cold, however, leaving you standing on the pedals, balancing. If so, lock both brakes, then push up and forward while releasing the brakes to ride up and out of the dip.

Pro Tip

How to Ride Safer in Wet Weather

FIRST: Don't let your wheels roll fully loaded over wet logs or rocks. Unweight each wheel as it touches the top of the obstacle by shifting your weight back, then forward.

SECOND: Make sure you have traction with the rear wheel. Spin a small gear so you keep momentum. You gain balance and traction from spinning wheels. Simply knowing you're good in wet conditions will give you an advantage over other riders. Maybe with some practice, you'll even learn to like rain and mud.

Parting the Waters

When you encounter a stream, dismounting and carrying your bike isn't always necessary. Four-time Leadville Trail 100 champ Laurie Brandt Hauptmann explains how to navigate shallow waterways.

SCOUT IT OUT

Most stream crossings are located at the bottom of a hill, so you'll probably approach fast. Slow down and determine where you'll enter and where you'll exit. Come to a complete stop if necessary. You can always back up and try it again after you have spied the line. Let your bike handling skills and environmental factors (i.e., don't trash a delicate bank) be your guides.

FIND A LINE

Avoid the direct line as often as you can. Why? Crossings that see frequent traffic, especially those shared with recreational off-road vehicles, will often have a pool that's been dug out right in the middle, with a treacherously soft bottom waiting like a pike to grab your wheels and toss you. I usually roll through the shallow riffle below the pool because I can see all the rocks and maneuver around them.

WATCH THE BOTTOM

Check out the bottom of the stream, too. You'll encounter everything from mud and sand to boulders and roots, and they're all slicker than

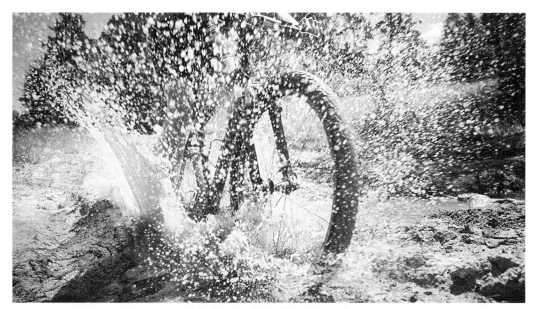
Pick a line, then let the bike do the work.

ice. Pebbles and small cobbles are easier to ride across (if they're not covered with slimy algae). When the rocks get bigger, picking a good line is harder. You might be able to weave through a rock garden on land, but it's considerably harder when the boulders are wet. In general, your knowledge of the area will help you discriminate. With extremely muddy or silty streams, it's sometimes better to wade through them.

MAKE THE CROSSING

Once you have determined the best line, build some momentum, shift to a gear that will enable you to accelerate in midstream if necessary, let go of the brakes, and go for it. Your goal is to get across by pedaling as little as possible—preferably not at all. Get into a low, crouched position out of the saddle, with your elbows and knees bent. Imitate a cat ready to pounce. Be light on the front wheel, with your weight slightly to the rear, as if you're descending. Make sure the crankarms are parallel to the water to keep your feet relatively dry and to give you the best chance of clearing rocks.

AFTER THE BATH

Good form will keep your head (and your bike) above water. Remember that once you've forded a stream, you still carry some of the stream with you. Mud or sand can make your tires slippery, so don't expect to arrive on the other side with the same traction you had going in. Ease into your dry-land pedaling—don't give a big power stroke as soon as you reach solid ground. It could be several minutes before your tires and rims dry out, so be conservative while braking and maneuvering until you know your rig has dried out. One last point: Before starting a ride that has many stream crossings, make sure your pedals are well lubed. Clipless pedals work best when the springs are covered with grease. Sure, sand and dirt will stick to them so they look like a lollipop dropped in a sandbox, but they're a lot safer. A dry pedal is a dangerous and unpredictable pedal. You don't want to get to the other side, grinning about your achievement, only to fall over because you can't release in a pinch.

How to Conquer Switchbacks

If you've ever ridden a singletrack with switchbacks, you'd know it. These turns curve back on themselves 180 degrees and are one of the toughest trail features for novice mountain bikers to master. Here's how to negotiate them.

BREATHE DEEPLY

About 10 to 20 feet before the switchback, take four or five deep breaths to get your body ready for increased effort.

SHIFT FOR SPIN AND TORQUE

You want a gear that's small enough to let you spin easily yet large enough to let you apply intense power to accelerate and ride up

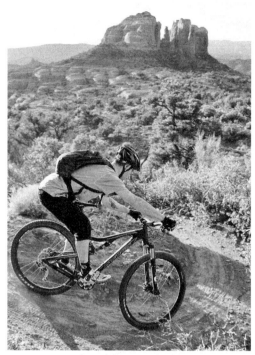

Look where you want the bike to go.

through the turn. Try a combo that feels slightly harder than you'd normally pick: the small chainring/third-from-largest cog works for most of us. *Bonus:* You're less likely to catch a pedal because you make fewer pedal strokes.

EYE THE EXIT

For smoother steering and better balance, your eyes should travel along your line before your bike does. Start from your front wheel, trace your planned line around the turn, then focus on an exit point 3 to 10 feet beyond the switchback. A common goof is fixating on your front wheel or even on the next 2 to 3 feet, which is hard to avoid on slow turns. Take your vision all the way around the switchback and out.

TAKE THE WIDE LINE

Don't follow the classic turn pattern (enter wide, go inside, exit wide)—that's the number one reason riders bite it. Your entire line should be in the outer half of the turn. The farther out, the better your traction. And the steeper the switchback, the farther out you should ride.

PEDAL AGAINST THE BRAKES

You will pedal more smoothly and have more control if you lightly drag both brakes. When you push easy gears in tight corners, your body has a tendency to bob disruptively on each downstroke. Dragging the brakes eliminates this weakness. You can also control the arc of your line: Tighten it by squeezing the brakes harder, widen it by easing off.

KEEP THE REAR IN LINE

Your wheels don't follow an identical line—the rear tire can track inside the front by a foot or more. Even though your front wheel rolls outside and clear, your rear wheel can butt against the steep, inside part of the apex and rob your momentum or stall you. Minimize the difference in the lines by steering with weight shifts instead of turning the handlebar.

RELAX

A lot of us tense up and stall at this point. Straight arms equal a tense rider. Flex your elbows. Breathe. Compare and contrast particle physics and string theory.

SWIVEL YOUR HIPS

To change direction without ratcheting the bar sideways, keep your butt on the saddle, your head centered, and use your hips to steer your bike through the turn. Make an arc with your hips and torso that follows the turn's curve: Start with your weight on the inside of the turn, then swing out and finally back in to finish the direction change. Confused? On a right-hand turn, your hips will trace a letter C as they move. For a left-hand turn, you'll trace a backward C.

DIP YOUR SHOULDER

Dip your inside shoulder a couple of inches to pull your bike into the turn. With your head slightly behind the axle, look through the exit and up the trail another 20 feet.

SLIDE YOUR BUTT FORWARD

Just past the apex, scoot forward on the saddle and bend closer to the bar. Shift your weight to the front wheel to compensate for the grade increase—but don't stand. Staying in contact with the saddle preserves the rear wheel's traction.

TURN FOR TRACTION

Once you've gotten the bike around the turn, you can turn the bar to avoid loose terrain or get more traction.

LEAN YOUR TORSO

To maintain traction, the angle of your lean over your bike should become sharper—from about 60 degrees to 45. As you climb the steep section after the turn, your nose should be over the stem.

Don't let tricky switchbacks intimidate you or slow you down. By practicing these tips, you'll learn to conquer the turns safely.

Surviving Your First Mountain Bike Race

The rarefied air and unending singletrack of Durango, Colorado, has produced some of America's best mountain bikers, including Daryl Price, a former pro. Though sometimes overshadowed by his neighbors John Tomac and Ned Overend, Price earned a reputation for consistency at the highest level of competition. Here's his advice on preparing for your first off-road race.

GET READY TO RACE

Keep in mind that nothing you do in the days just before the race will help you go faster in that race. It can only hurt you. In general I

start my preparation schedule 3 days out. On that day I just do 1 hour easy. The next day I ride the course and make a few spinning efforts up the climbs. That's at a real easy pace, for 1 or 2 hours, to get my legs moving and check out the course. The day before, I do 90 minutes on the course at a couple of notches below race speed. It needs to be a good tempo so I know how to set up for the corners and what the right line is. You need to learn the course.

CHECK YOUR EQUIPMENT

Check your equipment the day before, particularly tire pressure. If the course is rocky you need to run enough to prevent pinch flats. Also, a clean bike is a happy bike, so I try to wash it at night after I ride that day. I'll spray the bike, run a rag over it, and lubricate it. That means pulling the cables out of their stops and using a light oil on them, and oiling the chain. In general, try not to make too many adjustments—just tire and fork pressure. Don't do any equipment changes or derailleur adjustments. Those things will just create stress. Your bike should be dialed by then.

PREPARE FOR BREAKDOWNS

For the race I carry two CO_2 cartridges, a tube, and a multi-tool that includes a chain tool and 4, 5, and 6 mm Allen wrenches. I keep it all in a seat pack. I always carry this kit

SET YOUR SUSPENSION AND CHECK IT OFTEN

IT'S FRIGHTENING HOW MANY RIDERS HIT THE trail with poorly adjusted forks and shocks. Not only will a droopy suspension make your bike feel like a wet noodle, it can also be downright dangerous. A few simple adjustments are all it takes to have your suspension smoothly sucking up bumps.

Here are some general guidelines. Be sure to read the manufacturer's recommendations (found online or in your owner's manual), however, because they will provide the starting point based on your bike's suspension design. Because air can leak through the seals, remember to check your pressure monthly.

SAG: HOW MUCH THE SUSPENSION COMPRESSES WHEN YOU SIT ON THE BIKE

➤ For cross-country bikes: 20 to 25 percent of travel

➤ For trail bikes: 25 to 30 percent of travel

➤ For downhill bikes: 30 to 35 percent of travel

➤ For how to measure and set sag, visit Bicycling.com/video and search for "sag."

COMPRESSION: CONTROLS THE RATE AT WHICH THE SUSPENSION COMPRESSES IN RESPONSE TO A BUMP

➤ Start with the dial in the middle setting, and go ride.

➤ If the bike feels harsh, dial the damping down a click.

➤ If it feels mushy, add a click.

➤ Repeat until it feels smooth and supple.

REBOUND: THE RATE AT WHICH THE SUSPENSION RETURNS TO FULL EXTENSION)

➤ Again, start in the middle setting.

➤ Ride a short, rough section of trail. If the fork or shock seems too springy, add a click of rebound.

➤ If it bounces back too slowly, dial it back a click.

because I get paid to finish. I need as many series points as I can get, and if I don't have tools to fix my bike, it could cost me a national title. My sponsors pay a lot to get me to races, and I don't quit many of them.

WARM UP

I prefer to race in the morning because I can get nervous. Food doesn't settle, and you expend a lot of energy thinking about the race. Sometimes you need to go to the bathroom 10 times, even though you know you're not hydrated. In general, you have to try to relax. Don't tinker with your bike. Just lie there, stretch, watch some TV, and take in the calories.

Once you get to the course, do a 1-hour warm-up. Start with 30 minutes at a leisurely pace, then do 1- to 5-minute high-intensity efforts. You want to be on the line sweating, with your heart rate high.

STARTING

People coming from a road background find the start of mountain bike races to be ballistic. You sit at the start for 15 minutes, then your heart rate goes from 80 to 180 instantly. Everyone's legs feel like cement. It's super high-intensity, and then you just go until you fade. That's basically what a mountain bike race is. So instead of experiencing the start for the first time in a race, ensure that you can go at a high intensity by doing it in training.

The effort you put in at the start also depends on what the course is like. Some narrow to singletrack quickly, and the position you have going into it is the position you'll have coming out. If you're in 30th going in you'll be at least a minute behind, and it will be hard to do well. When the course narrows to singletrack, people lose their marbles. People who were your friends are suddenly fighting you for 25th place. If there's more doubletrack on the course you can pace yourself into the start. That means riding the wheels in front of you, but not fighting for them as much.

PACING

Treat the race like a time trial. Just go your max. You can pace yourself and catch people who are dying later on, but it's better to go hard from the start. You can also make a special effort on certain sections. For instance, if I'm behind Dave Wiens on a sketchy downhill, I'll try to get by beforehand. And I'll pass Bob Roll before a singletrack section. But I'll follow John Tomac anywhere. Ned Overend, too. They're good on anything. But certain people I'll race into a part of the course.

I also wear a heart rate monitor, but mostly just to recall the information on a computer afterward. I'll look at it sometimes in a race. I'll never slow if it tells me my heart rate is high (around 190). On the other hand, if I see it's 170, I know I can do 15 bpm more, so I might go harder.

REFUEL WHILE RACING

I usually drink one bottle of energy drink and have one bottle handed to me during the race. And I have water in a second bottle. I don't use solid food—it's impossible in a mountain bike race. You can hardly drink, much less eat. It's hard to take your hands off the bar.

COOL DOWN

It's a good idea to warm down with some easy pedaling after the race, but usually it's unrealistic. You're so tired. First, get clean and get a bottle. Then reward yourself. If you want a soda, have a soda. That night, if you want a beer, have one. That's what it's all about. Reward yourself. Get two scoops of ice cream. You have to enjoy the event to the same degree that you sacrificed for it.

Training Plan

When you blast beyond the bounds of your aerobic fitness, your technical skills take a dive. This plan builds base fitness while honing your top speed. Try to do at least half of the interval sessions on dirt.

WORKOUTS

All rides are at a conversational pace (easy to moderate) on flat to rolling terrain, unless otherwise noted.

ACTIVE RECOVERY: Easy ride, light gear, moderate cadence

CLIMB REPEATS: Steady climb at 78 to 83 percent of maximum heart rate, cadence 70 to 85 rpm

ENDURANCE: Ride at this level (zone 2) to build a base of endurance and enhance your aerobic fitness

STEADY STATE: A longer effort at your lactate threshold (85 percent + 3 bpm of your maximum heart rate), cadence 85 to 95 rpm

HILL ACCELERATIONS: Pedal normally until the final 500 yards of the hill, then gradually accelerate to nearly reach your maximum heart rate; start the interval the last few yards of the hill, out of the saddle at max effort

POWER INTERVALS: Pace above lactate threshold with a perceived exertion of 8 to 9, or 90 to 95 percent of your maximum heart rate

TEMPO: Work at 80 percent of your maximum heart rate in a larger gear, cadence 70 to 75 rpm

MAXIMUM VO$_2$ INTERVALS: Work as hard as possible, paying no attention to heart rate, to boost your maximum oxygen consumption (max VO$_2$) levels

HILL SPRINTS: An all-out sprint on a hill

Think you're ready to tackle a mountain bike stage race? Visit Bicycling.com/mtbstagerace.

Mountain Bike Training Plan

WEEK	MONDAY	TUESDAY	WEDNESDAY	THURSDAY	FRIDAY	SATURDAY	SUNDAY
1	Rest day	**END** with 3 × 10-min Climb Repeats; 10 min rest 1 hr, 30 min	Rest day	**END** with 3 × 8-min Climb Repeats; 8 min rest 1 hr, 30 min	Rest day	**END** 2 hr, 30 min	**END** 2 hr
2	Rest day	**END** with 3 × 12-min Climb Repeats; 10 min rest 1 hr, 45 min	Rest day	**END** with 3 × 10-min Climb Repeats; 8 min rest 1 hr, 45 min	Rest day	**END** 2 hr, 45 min	**END** 2 hr, 30 min
3	Rest day	**END** with 3 × 15-sec Hill Accelerations; 3 min rest 1 hr, 45 min	Rest day	**END** with 3 × 6-min Climb Repeats; 6 min rest 1 hr, 45 min	Rest day	**END** with 2 sets of 2 × 3-min Power Intervals; 3 min rest; 6 min between sets 3 hr, 30 min	**END** 2 hr, 45 min
4	Rest day	**END** 1 hr	Rest day	**END** 1 hr, 30 min	Rest day	**END** 2 hr, 30 min	**END** with 30-min Tempo 2 hr, 30 min
5	Rest day	**END** with 2 sets of 3 × 3-min Power Intervals; 3 min rest; 8 min between sets 1 hr, 30 min	Rest day	**END** with 2 sets of 2 × 3-min. Power Intervals; 3 min rest; 8 min between sets 1 hr, 30 min	Rest day	**END** with 3 × 3-min Power Intervals; 10 min rest 2 hr, 30 min	**END** with 3 × 10-min Steady State; 10 min rest 2 hr, 30 min
6	Rest day	**END** with 3 sets of 3 × 3-min Power Intervals; 3 min rest; 6 min between sets 1 hr, 30 min	Rest day	**END** with 4 × 6-min Climb Repeats; 6 min rest 1 hr, 30 min	Rest day	**END** with 2 sets of 2 × 4-min Power Intervals; 4 min rest; 10 min between sets 2 hr, 30 min	**END** with 3 × 15-sec Hill Accelerations; 3 min rest 2 hr, 45 min
7	Rest day	**END** with 4 × 30-sec Max VO_2 intervals; 30 sec rest 2 hr	Rest day	**END** with 4 × 8-min Climb Repeats; 8 min rest 1 hr, 45 min	Rest day	**END** with 6 ×10-sec Hill Sprints; 5 min rest 2 hr, 45 min	**END** 3 hr
8	Rest day	**END** 1 hr	Rest day	**END** with 20-min Tempo 1 hr, 30 min	Rest day	**END** 2 hr	**END** with 30-min Tempo 3 hr

Abbreviations: END, endurance/zone 2; max VO_2, maximum VO_2/zone 5; tempo, zone 3.

WEEK	MONDAY	TUESDAY	WEDNESDAY	THURSDAY	FRIDAY	SATURDAY	SUNDAY
9	Rest day	**END** with 2 sets of 3 × 3-min Power Intervals; 3 min rest; 8 min between sets 2 hr	Rest day	**END** with 3 × 6-min Climb Repeats; 6 min rest 2 hr	Rest day	**END** with 4 × 3-min Power Intervals; 4 min rest 3 hr	**END** 2 hr, 30 min
10	Rest day	**END** with 3 sets of 4 × 30-sec Max VO$_2$ Intervals; 30 sec rest; 8 min between sets 1 hr, 30 min	Rest day	**END** with 2 sets of 3 × 3-min Power Intervals; 3 min rest; 8 min between sets 1 hr, 45 min	Rest day	**END** with 45-min Tempo 2 hr	**END** 2 hr, 30 min
11	Rest day	**END** with 5 × 10-sec Hill Sprints; 5 min rest 1 hr, 45 min	Rest day	**END** with 3 × 2-min Power Intervals; 2 min rest 1 hr, 30 min	Rest day	**END** with 45-min Tempo 2 hr	**END** 2 hr, 30 min
12	Rest day	**END** with 2 sets of 5 × 30-sec Max VO$_2$ Intervals; 30 sec rest; 8 min between sets 1 hr, 30 min	Rest day	**Active Recovery** 1 hr	Rest day	**END** with 3 × 2-min Power Intervals; 5 min rest 1 hr	Race day

PART V

TEND

Training and racing is hard. It breaks your body down only to build it back up again. Sometimes, despite your best efforts, pounds pile on, fatigue accumulates, and injuries occur. To survive this punishing but ultimately rewarding—we swear!—cycle, you'll need to commit to performing regular maintenance. Consider these chapters your guide to achieving your ideal weight, mastering recovery, and attending to nagging aches and pains.

CHAPTER 14

Your Ideal Cycling Weight

I get embarrassed when I see how slim I was.

—Eddy Merckx, Belgian five-time Tour de France winner

BEHOLD THE MIGHTY POUND. EACH ONE HAS POTENTIAL: TO put raw power into your pedals. To outsprint the masses to the line. To ascend the likes of Mont Ventoux. Pack on too many pounds, however—especially the non-power-producing variety (in other words, fat)—and they'll weigh you down, slow you down, and maybe even shorten your life. Shave off too many, and you risk losing some of your crank-churning power. That's why, of all the figures cyclists track, from heart rate to mileage to speed, perhaps none outrank the one on the bathroom scale.

"I spend a lot of time helping riders achieve their ideal weight because the rewards are so great," says Hunter Allen, founder of the Peaks Coaching Group and coauthor of *Training and Racing with a Power Meter*. "Every extra pound you carry above that weight makes you 15 to 20 seconds slower for each mile of a climb." Off the bike, the rewards are just as substantial. The Centers for Disease Control and Prevention reports that losing just 5 to 10 percent of your total body weight can lower your blood pressure, improve cholesterol levels, and protect against diabetes and cancer. Even if you never compete, slimming down will help you enjoy riding more because your heart won't have to work as hard. Maybe you'll even drop some of those leaner-than-thou types on the group ride. You get the idea.

This is about being strong, not skinny. Fat plays a key role in immune system function: If you don't have enough fat, your energy will flag and you'll get sick. Become so lean that you start to burn muscle, and your power will plummet. The idea is to find a sweet spot where you can ride strong yet be healthy, too.

This sweet spot depends on numerous factors, including your current weight, height, and body frame size. In this section, we give you three ways to reach a target ideal weight in which you can live, ride, or even race for life. Focus on the method that best fits your goals, or try all three. Then read ahead for our training plan and nutrition suggestions designed to help you achieve your ideal cycling weight—and stay there for good.

What's your ideal cycling weight? Find out using the self-assessments on these pages.

Note: These formulas and plans are not a substitute for medical advice. Consult with a physician before embarking on any weight-loss program.

Option 1: Shed Excess Pounds

If you fit one or more of the descriptions below, use the steps in Option 1 to estimate an ideal target weight for your height and body frame size.

—You ride a few times a week, primarily for recreation.

—You used to ride all the time, and maybe even raced, but work, family, and other responsibilities have forced you to scale back.

—You know you've got some weight to lose before you can think about improving your performance on the bike.

STEP 1: FIND YOUR BASELINE HEALTHY WEIGHT

Use the following formula to find your baseline healthy weight:

MEN: 106 pounds for first 5 feet of height plus 6 pounds for each additional inch. For example, if you're 5'10'', your ideal weight is 166 pounds (106 + 60).

WOMEN: 100 pounds for the first 5 feet of height plus 5 pounds for each additional inch. For example, if you're 5'6'', your ideal weight is 130 pounds (100 + 30).

Baseline target weight (from step 1): _____ pounds

STEP 2: FACTOR IN YOUR FRAME SIZE

Just as mountain bikes come in small, medium, and large, so do our skeletal frames. That's why there's a range of medically recommended weights for any given height. A standard measurement of frame size is your wrist circumference in relation to your height. Use a tape measure to measure your wrist in inches at its widest point, then locate your frame size in this chart. Match your wrist size to your height:

WRIST			
MEN*: HEIGHT > 5'5"	5.5 to 6.5"	6.5"–7.5"	> 7.5"
WOMEN: HEIGHT < 5'2"	< 5.5'	5.5"–5.75"	> 5.75"
WOMEN: HEIGHT 5'2"–5'5"	< 6"	6"–6.25"	> 6.25"
WOMEN: HEIGHT > 5'5"	< 6.25"	6.25"–6.5"	> 6.5"
FRAME SIZE	Small	Medium	Large

*Women vary more by height and frame size than men do and therefore have more variation in this ratio.

If your frame size is:

SMALL: Subtract 10 percent from your baseline target weight

MEDIUM: Keep your baseline target weight

LARGE: Add 10 percent to your baseline target weight

Target ideal weight (from step 2): _____ pounds

This number is your adjusted target weight. Standard body weight formulas are based on averages, which means that results for some people may be slightly skewed. If the number you calculate is equal to or greater than your current weight, or if it's too low to be attainable, try the formula in Option 2, which focuses on your body composition.

Option 2: Get Leaner and Faster

If you fit one or more of the descriptions below, use the following steps to estimate a weight that will maximize your body composition.

—You ride 4 or more days a week, including hard-charging training rides.

—You want to be competitive in a gran fondo, do a hard century, or race occasionally.

—You want to maximize your body composition and gain more power.

—The target ideal weight you calculated in Option 1 is greater than your current weight.

Body composition is a set of percentages that breaks down your weight into fat and lean pedal-pushing muscle. You'll get the most accurate reading from a special body composition scale. (You can buy these devices, which are also found in most fitness centers.) To get the most precise reading, make sure you use or purchase one that takes into account fitness level and follow the directions carefully.

The reading is sensitive to your hydration level and, for women, menstrual cycles. Like your weight, the figure will fluctuate, so try to calculate your average numbers over a couple of weeks. Avoid online calculators; they don't provide accurate readings for active people.

Your current body fat: ____ percent

Healthy body fat ranges are 10 to 25 percent for men and 18 to 30 percent for women (who naturally have more fat). Athletes in top form may fall below these numbers. If your body fat percentage is higher, decide on a goal number within the healthy range. Be realistic and don't just target the lowest possible percentage. "Having a bit more body fat is better for your immune system and for consistency on the bike," Allen says.

Your body fat goal: ____ percent

Follow these steps to come up with an ideal weight based on body composition.

STEP 1

Figure out how many pounds of body fat you have:

Your current weight × your body fat percentage
= ____ pounds
(EXAMPLE: 200 pounds × .28 = 56 pounds)

STEP 2

Next, figure out your lean body mass:

Your current weight - pounds of body fat
= ____ pounds
(EXAMPLE: 200 - 56 = 144 pounds)

STEP 3

Now, subtract your goal body fat percentage from 1.00.

1.00 - your goal body fat percentage
= ____ **(EXAMPLE:** 1.00 - .20 = .80)

STEP 4

Divide your lean body mass from Step 2 by your answer in Step 3 (**EXAMPLE:** 144 pounds / .80 = 180 pounds).

Your answer = ____ pounds

This is your target ideal weight based on body composition.

Option 3:
Get Competitive

If you fit one or more of the descriptions below, use the following guidelines to figure out how your weight compares with riders at cycling's highest levels.

—You are a competitive racer who trains 10 to 15 hours a week.

—You're already lean, but you aspire to achieve a racing weight comparable to that of the fastest racers.

—Your body fat is at the low end of the healthy range (or lower).

CAUTION: This weight may not be realistic or even healthy to maintain long-term. For many cyclists, these numbers may be aggressively low. Unless you get really serious about racing, you might want to set your sights a little higher.

Cycling coach Joe Friel, creator of the Training Bible series of books, has calculated that top male riders generally carry 2.1 to 2.4 pounds per inch and top women come in at 1.9 to 2.2 pounds per inch. That means a 5′10″ man would weigh 147 to 168 pounds and a 5′5″ woman would tip the scales between 123 and 143. Elite climbing specialists are often even lighter. Extra weight exacts far less of a penalty on flat ground than it does when you head toward the heavens on 10 percent grades. (This ratio isn't the same as your power-to-weight ratio, which is considered the gold standard for determining your most competitive cycling weight. It's close, however, and it doesn't require an expensive power meter to figure out.)

There are exceptions, says Friel. Even a cursory glance at the others in your cycling club will tell you that fast, successful riders come in all sizes. Riders like Cadel Evans are just built bigger than Andy and Fränk Schleck, but that doesn't make them slower. If you tend toward the muscular side, it can be unrealistic, if not downright counterproductive, to try to achieve an unnaturally low weight.

Use Friel's ranges above to see how close your goal or current weight is to a weight that would maximize your ability to compete (assuming you have the corresponding fitness). If your goal or current weight is less than your competitive weight, go back to Option 2 to make sure your body fat is within a healthy range. If it's not, hit the gym to put on lean muscle tissue and be sure you're properly fueling during and especially after your rides, so you don't go into a catabolic state and eat into your precious muscle stores. Be especially sure to meet your daily protein requirements by including it in every meal and snack.

Ride It Off: Your Quick-Start Plan

Now that you know what you want to weigh, it's time to plot how to get there. The following 2-week plan from coach Hunter Allen will jump-start your weight loss by training your body to become a fat-burning machine. "It combines intense efforts with on-bike fueling strategies to teach your body to burn fat more effectively," he says. "It's not about drilling it every day. It's about becoming a strong, well-rounded rider and an excellent fat burner." You'll get noticeable results fast.

HOW IT WORKS

The program assumes you hop on your bike (or a stationary bike at the gym) 4 or more days a week. If you've been riding less than that, take the easy days as full rest and begin with the fewest number of intervals indicated on a given day.

Keep your calorie intake in check by limiting snacks on easy and rest days. On days that include hills, intervals, and/or other hard work right after your warm-up, have a preride snack. For endurance rides (days 6, 7, 13, and 14), when you'll pedal at a lower intensity, roll out the door on an empty stomach, ideally in the morning before breakfast or a few hours after a meal later in the day. Take plenty of food with you for on-bike snack suggestions. You can fuel up after the 90-minute mark before you drain your glycogen stores and bonk. "The idea is to train your body to become an efficient fat burner while still properly fueling your ride," Allen says. At first, it may be difficult to wait this long to start eating. Remember to ride at an easy to moderate effort. You should be able to carry on a conversation easily. If you're really flagging, have a bite or two at the 1-hour mark and extend from there on subsequent rides.

Day 1

Lengthen your planned ride by 30 minutes and add one to three 10-minute intervals at an effort close to what you could maintain in a 60-minute time trial, or a rate of perceived exertion (see below) of 5 on a scale of 1 to 10. Pedal lightly for 5 minutes between each interval.

Day 2

Include two to five 3-minute intervals in your planned ride, maintaining the hardest steady effort you can. Pedal lightly for 3 minutes between each interval.

Day 3

Lengthen your planned ride by adding 45 minutes, structured as one 8- to 10-second sprint every 2 minutes at 80 percent of your all-out effort (rate of perceived exertion 8). Maintain a moderate to somewhat strong effort in between sprints (rate of perceived exertion 3 to 4).

RATE OF PERCEIVED EXERTION (RPE)

0 Very Easy	**5** Strong
1 to 2 Easy	**6 to 7** Very strong
3 Moderate	**8** Extremely strong
4 Somewhat strong	**9 to 10** All-out

Day 4

Include 5 to 10 1-minute intervals in your planned ride. Do these aggressively (rate of perceived exertion 7 to 8) and attack so that you're fading (but still pushing) in the final 15 seconds. Pedal lightly for 2 minutes between each.

Day 5

Spin easy for an hour or take a rest day.

Day 6

Endurance ride. Aim for 2 hours at an easy to moderate effort (rate of perceived exertion 2 to 3). If you haven't done a ride of this length recently, extend your longest recent ride by one-third.

Day 7

Endurance ride. Aim for 3 hours at an easy to moderate effort (rate of perceived exertion 2 to 3), or extend your longest recent ride by one-third.

Day 8

Spin easy for an hour or take a rest day.

Day 9

Include two to four 10-minute intervals in your regular ride at an effort close to what you could maintain in a 60-minute time trial (rate of perceived exertion 5). Push yourself hard during the last 2 minutes. Pedal lightly to recover for 5 minutes between each interval.

Day 10

Include 5 to 10 15-second all-out sprints (rate of perceived exertion 10) in your regular ride. Pedal lightly to recover for 4 minutes between each. Alternate between small- and big-ring sprints.

Day 11

Include the following anaerobic intervals in a regular ride: three 2-minute intervals at rate of perceived exertion 7 with 2 minutes of easy pedaling between each. Ride 5 minutes easy. Then do three 1-minute intervals at rate of perceived exertion 8 with 1 minute of recovery in between. Ride 5 minutes easy and finish with three 30-second intervals, going all-out, with 1 minute of easy pedaling in between.

Day 12

Lengthen your regular ride by 45 minutes today and pedal that final stretch at nearly your time trial pace, or upper-tempo pace (rate of perceived exertion 4).

Day 13

Endurance ride. Aim for 2.5 to 3 hours, easy to moderate effort (rate of perceived exertion 2 to 3), or extend your longest recent ride by one-third.

Day 14

Long endurance ride. Plan to pedal for 3 to 4 hours at an easy to moderate effort (rate of perceived exertion 2 to 3), or extend your longest recent ride by one-third.

Eat Smart, Go Faster

Though some people have an easier time slimming down than others, weight loss is basically about how many calories you eat versus how many you burn. Here's the simple math: One pound equals 3,500 calories. To lose a pound a week, create a daily deficit of 500 calories by eating less and/or burning more. The biggest challenge for a cyclist is to create this deficit while still getting enough fuel to sustain your rides. "This is where the timing of your calories—and their composition—becomes essential," says Anne Guzman, sports nutrition consultant for Peaks Coaching Group. It's also where most of us get it wrong.

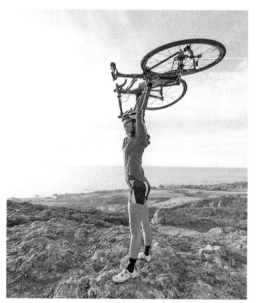

Get lean without sacrificing strength. It's possible.

Some riders try to lose weight by underfueling their rides. This always backfires. "If you don't eat enough on the bike, you'll empty your stored glycogen, forcing your body to break down muscle tissue for energy," Guzman says. If you start depleting muscle, your performance suffers. It does no good to be skinny if you're too weak to keep up. Chances are you won't get skinny, because you'll finish the ride starving and eat everything in sight. It's more effective to eat measured portions of the right kinds of calories throughout the day. Don't devalue carbs: Although protein is vital for muscle repair, carbs are a cyclist's primary source of fuel during training, Guzman says.

Based on these principles, Guzman created an eating program based on whole foods with high nutritional value that will optimize your health and weight. Each meal provides a balance of slow-burning carbs to fuel your riding, muscle-mending protein, healthy fat for energy and immunity, and an array of fruits and vegetables.

For rides less than 90 minutes, Guzman recommends electrolyte drinks; for longer rides, look for energy drinks that are 4 to 7 percent carbohydrates. Otherwise, reach for flavored waters, coffee, tea, and other low-sugar, low-calorie drinks. Avoid soda, fruit juices, and diet soft drinks (artificial sweeteners have been linked to fat gain). Alcohol delivers empty calories and, while a glass of

POWER-TO-WEIGHT RATIO

THE SINGLE BEST MEASURE OF YOUR CYCLING performance is your power-to-weight ratio. This figure refers to the maximum power output measured in watts that you can sustain for an extended period of time, generally 30 minutes or more. You'll need a power meter to find this number.

The standard test for determining power is to perform a 20-minute time trial on an uphill grade. No hill at your disposal? Simulate the test on a flat road or trainer. Avoid rolling roads, which will lower your overall power number. Record the average wattage you produce, then divide the watts by your morning body weight in kilograms (pounds divided by 2.2). So if you weigh 180 pounds (82 kilograms) and you average 270 watts, your power-to-weight ratio is 3.3 watts per kilogram.

To score a top spot on the Trek Factory Racing pro team, that number would need to be above 6 watts per kilogram. Beginner cyclists usually pull in the range of 2.5 to 3.2 for men and 2.1 to 2.8 for women. Fast recreational riders produce wattage in the range of 3.7 to 4.4 for men and 3.2 to 3.8 for women.

If you're cranking out 2.9 and want to hit 3.9, look at your weight first. If it's not optimal, use our weight-loss training and nutrition plans. If it's where you want it to be, work on your power. Regular strength training, especially squats, leg presses, and step-ups, can do the job.

wine with dinner isn't a crime, if you want to get lean, consider how those calories fit into your daily total. As for sweets, it's okay to splurge on dessert now and then.

Stay Lean for Life

Anyone who has ever been on a diet knows that dropping pounds turns out to be the easy part. Keeping them off? Not so much. In fact, a recent study puts the odds at one in six for maintaining weight loss. That's pretty discouraging news. The better news is that as an active cyclist, you're already one step ahead of the game. "People who maintain their activity levels have much better odds of staying at their lower weight," says Leslie Bonci, MPH, RD, director of sports nutrition at the

DOES BODY SHAPE MATTER?

MOST OF US CAN SLOT OUR OVERALL build into one of three general categories. Which type are you?

ECTOMORPH

YOU TEND TO HAVE LONG LIMBS AND a small frame. Your muscles are lean and sinewy, not bulky, and you may have trouble keeping weight on. To gain strength and lean muscle mass, work your large muscle groups with squats and leg presses and by performing big-gear intervals on the bike. Be sure to get enough protein by including it in every meal.

MESOMORPH

YOU'RE NATURALLY MUSCULAR AND PROPORTIONALLY BUILT AND tend toward the lean side. While you shouldn't seek to deliberately lose muscle, you may want to avoid gaining it where you don't need it for cycling, like on your upper body.

ENDOMORPH

YOU ARE GENERALLY MORE HEAVYSET, ESPECIALLY AROUND your midsection, and have a hard time losing fat. Even though muscle is an athlete's engine, too much can weigh you down. Try plyometrics (see Chapter 5) to improve the speed and force of your muscle contractions without increasing bulk.

University of Pittsburgh Medical Center and author of *The Active Calorie Diet.*

The National Weight Control Registry reports that among people who successfully keep weight off, men burn an average of 3,293 calories a week and women an average of 2,545. That works out to about an hour of moderate riding every day. As activity levels slide, weight creeps back on.

You may also need to start eating a little less, because losing weight resets your metab-olism. Plus, the more you ride, the more effi-cient you become at burning calories. In short, the new, leaner you needs fewer calories to sustain your body both on and off your bike. The adjustments aren't huge. For each pound you lose, your total daily calorie requirements dip by about 10. So a rider who dropped 10 pounds needs 100 fewer calories each day. Keep following the plan until you hit your goal weight. Then stay with it for 3 months, allow-ing your metabolism to adjust.

Having a focused plan can also help. Here are four other strategies that researchers have linked to keeping weight off.

1. **EAT BREAKFAST:** It keeps your energy level steady so you don't overeat later in the day.

2. **WEIGH IN:** The vast majority of people who stay slim step on a scale at least once a week—those concrete numbers staring up at you are simply too hard to ignore.

3. **BE CONSISTENT:** Most folks who keep the pounds off do so by staying the course. They eat well most of the time without swinging between deprivation and bingeing.

4. **REWARD YOURSELF:** Giving yourself strategic incentives for healthy behavior can prevent backsliding. Choose health incentives, such as a new jersey or gloves, rather than unhealthy options like, say, cake.

CHAPTER 15

Recovery

You've got to rest as hard as you train.

—ROGER YOUNG, US NATIONAL TRACK SPRINT CHAMPION
AND OLYMPIC GOLD MEDALIST

THOUGH HE SPENDS THOUSANDS OF HOURS ON THE BIKE, SOME of Chris Horner's most important race prep takes place on the couch. "It's a physical and mental break," says the team Lampre-Merida pro, about getting off his feet and paying attention to his remote instead of his watts.

Plenty of everyday cyclists log far fewer miles than Horner, yet they still risk injury, overtraining, and burnout by neglecting this kind of downtime. "They think they can't afford to go easy," says Stephen Cheung, PhD, a professor of kinesiology at Brock University in St. Catherines, Ontario, and coauthor of *Cutting-Edge Cycling*. "But recovery is just as valuable as training, if not more so."

One of the ways you become a better cyclist is through muscular adaptation. In very basic terms, this is what happens: The stress of training causes small tears in your muscles. Your body then repairs the damage, which results in an inflammatory response (the swelling and tenderness you feel after a hard workout or race). This rebuilding process creates stronger muscles, but only if the body has adequate time to heal. "If you start your next ride when you're not completely recovered," says Max Testa, MD, chief medical officer for Team BMC and former team doctor for 7-Eleven and Motorola, "your body's at a disadvantage and you'll grow more tired and gain less from each workout."

Recovery isn't just about sitting on the couch with your legs up. It's also about not going hard all the time and using days off wisely. Strategies like low-intensity rides and massage allow your muscles to benefit from all the work you've put in. Here's how to maximize every minute you spend in—and out—of the saddle.

When to Recover

Before you wrap yourself in compression wear and guzzle chocolate milk after every ride, make sure your effort warrants it. If you didn't go hard enough to induce muscle fiber damage and suck your energy stores dry, you might not need full-on recovery, says coach Hunter Allen. If your ride meets any of the descriptions in the box "Recover If You Rode . . ." you could probably benefit from some R & R. Try some of the tried-and-true techniques below.

Rest, Actively

In a well-thought-out training plan, rest usually doesn't mean doing nothing. In fact, many coaches prefer low-effort workouts to total rest on off or easy days to get blood circulating and reduce inflammation so you're primed for your next ride.

Another form of active rest is the post-ride cool down at the end of a long or hard effort.

RECOVER IF YOU RODE...

➤ 2 hours or less with at least 20 minutes at maximum effort

➤ 2.5 hours with at least 30 minutes very hard

➤ 2.5-plus hours with at least 40 minutes hard

➤ 4-plus hours with at least 40 minutes moderately hard

BUT, WAIT: ISN'T INFLAMMATION GOOD?

YOU MIGHT BE WONDERING WHY YOU SHOULD limit inflammation if it ultimately helps muscles grow stronger. Some inflammation is good when training, says Testa, but you don't want so much inflammation that you're too sore or tired to ride. The muscle-soothing, injury-preventing effects of simple recovery methods can help you face your next hard ride fresh and ready to go. Especially if you're doing a stage race or a multiday or century ride, it's critical to wake up feeling capable of more miles, according to Testa. It's the main reason Tour de France riders put in 2 to 3 hours in the saddle on rest days.

Easing up on the pedals enhances blood flow to help flush your legs of lactic acid and fuel your depleted muscles. A study in the *Journal of Strength and Conditioning Research* found that when cyclists did a 15-minute cool down spin at 30 percent of their maximum VO_2 after a hard effort, they were able to perform almost as well 24 hours later on an identical strenuous workout.

DO IT: Plan active recovery workouts for the day after a high-mileage weekend, a hard interval session, or a race. For these rides, the trick is to go deliberately—borderline embarrassingly—slow. Cheung describes it as "letting-your-grandmother-beat-you" easy. You don't have to limit yourself to the bike: Walking, easy swimming, or light jogging count. As for a cool down, dial your effort back to a "pedal-to-the-coffee-shop" intensity during the last 5 to 10 minutes of

your ride, says Cheung. Keep power and resistance low, heart rate slightly elevated.

GET A MASSAGE

A post-ride rubdown helps increase circulation and clear muscles of lactic acid, says Reed McCalvin, personal soigneur to Taylor Phinney. It also reduces adhesions, or knots, that make movement less efficient and more painful. What's more, science has linked massage to improved muscle function. In a study on cyclists who got a massage on only one leg, biopsies showed greater muscle regeneration in the treated leg. Researchers in Canada have also found that massage after exercise reduced inflammation and promoted the growth of new mitochondria, the parts of your cells that produce power.

There's also a mental benefit to massage, says Testa. Numerous studies have shown that it lowers levels of the stress hormone cortisol, which is released during hard efforts. "If your brain remains in fighting mode," says Testa, "it slows your recovery." Excess cortisol has been linked to overtraining syndrome and can lead to a host of problems, including irritability, weight gain, and muscle loss.

DO IT: No soigneur on your payroll? You can buy a foam roller at most sporting goods stores and use it after a ride or anytime in between. Rest your leg muscles and glutes on the cylinder and roll slowly back and forth, pausing and pressing into the sorest spots for 30 to 45 seconds. For hard-to-reach areas, such as shoulder blades and other parts of your back, lean against a tennis ball on the wall. See page 93 for six foam roller moves.

TAKE A COLD PLUNGE

Long a favorite ritual of distance runners, soaking in cold water after a workout has been shown to reduce inflammation and soreness. The same *Journal of Strength and Conditioning Research* study previously mentioned found that a group of cyclists who immersed their legs in cold water right after a hard effort performed even better on a second rigorous ride 24 hours later. Another benefit: Soaking in cold water can simply feel good, especially on hot days. Whether it leads to actual strength gains is up for debate. A recent review of 17 studies found that while it does reduce pain,

cold-water immersion might not make muscles stronger.

DO IT: Fill a tub with about 8 inches of 50° to 60°F water. This should be enough water to cover your legs while you're in a seated position. Soak for up to 15 minutes within a half hour of finishing a hard ride. If you can't tolerate the chill, start with shorter baths and try keeping your shorts on and wearing a fleece jacket.

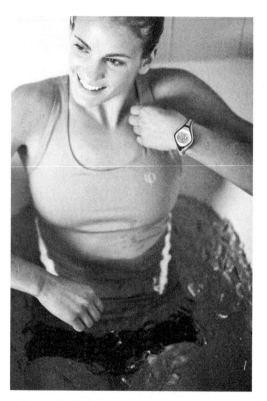

To ease the shock, submerge your legs in a tub of cool water, *then* add ice.

REFUEL THE RIGHT WAY

At the end of Tour de France stages in the mid-1980s, 7-Eleven team members would immediately drink soda to spike insulin stores, says Testa. They'd then eat a sandwich, yogurt with fruit, and maybe some cheese with potatoes later at the hotel. These days, team directors use a more formulaic approach: Riders guzzle recovery drinks with an ideal balance of muscle-mending protein and glycogen-replacing carbohydrates that are easy to digest and quickly enter the system.

DO IT: Unless you're pressed for time, it's easy enough to get these nutrients from real food. The optimal formula is four parts carbohydrate and one part protein. Good post-ride recovery snacks include a smoothie made with Greek yogurt, a banana, and berries or a bowl of cereal with fruit and milk, says sports nutritionist Nancy Clark, RD. For a meal, try a turkey and cheese sandwich or spaghetti and meatballs made with turkey or lean beef.

You also need to replace sodium and potassium lost through sweat and, while commercial sports drinks are handy, says Clark, low-fat milk (regular or chocolate) and other convenient foods, such as pretzels, a bagel with peanut butter, or pasta with tomato sauce, can be even better for replacing these electrolytes—and for your overall health.

As for timing, feed muscles as quickly as possible after a workout, especially if you have less than 24 hours until your next hard effort. "Within 15 to 30 minutes is ideal," says Testa. Try to eat something else in the next 60 to 90 minutes, when your body's primed to take in nutrients and replenish energy stores. No matter how exhausted you are at the end of a long day, topping off the tank before heading to bed may help repair muscles while you're down for the count. In a study published in *Medicine and Science in Sports and Exercise*, researchers had one group of exercisers drink a protein shake 30 minutes before bed and another group a shake without protein. Overnight muscle-protein synthesis rates were 22 percent higher in the protein drinkers.

SLEEP MORE

It's well known that pro cyclists sleep far more than the average club rider, clocking up to 70 hours of shut-eye a week during the Tour de France, for example, compared with the 40 to 50 hours most of us get during the same time period. It's a recovery tool that pro teams take seriously for good reason: When you sleep, your body produces hormones that are critical to recovery. Research has shown that getting just 2 fewer hours of sleep than normal can slow your reaction time. Indeed, it can be a key factor in athletic performance, says Stanford University sleep researcher Cheri Mah, MS, but one we often neglect. In 2011, Mah and her colleagues found that when athletes who were sleeping 6 to 8 hours a night aimed to get closer to 10 hours, their reaction time and performance improved. To get more sleep at night, stick to these nine golden rules.

1. **KEEP RIDING:** But try not to exercise within 4 hours of bedtime, says sleep expert Michael Breus, PhD. Exercise raises your body temperature, which triggers a shutdown of the sleep hormone melatonin. Also watch for signs of overtraining. If you feel crappy every time you get on the bike, consider taking some time off.

2. **AIM FOR 7 TO 9 HOURS:** That's what the body needs to cycle through the restorative phases of sleep.

3. **STICK TO A SCHEDULE:** "The more your body clock is locked in, the better," says Breus. Yes, you may be more sensitive to sleep disruptions, but Christopher Winter, MD, medical director of the Martha Jefferson Sleep Medicine Center in Charlottesville, Virginia, says that having a set schedule also makes you better equipped to handle them.

4. **EMBRACE THE DARK:** Darkness stimulates melatonin production. That means lights out when you're trying to sleep (no TV, laptop, or phone). I now put a small beanbag pillow over my eyes to block the light.

Breus also suggests I set the sleep timer on my TV so it's not running all night.

5. **STAY COOL:** Keep your bedroom between 65 and 75 degrees, say Breus. Any warmer and your body will think it's time to wake up.

6. **MANAGE CAFFEINE:** You don't have to sacrifice the performance benefits of caffeine. "But cut it off by 2 p.m.," Breus says. "It stays in your body for 8 to 10 hours after you drink it." Limit your intake to less than 250 milligrams a day, which is roughly the amount in two espressos, 21 ounces of sports drink, a 12-ounce soda, or an energy gel.

7. **CURTAIL BOOZE FOR 3 HOURS BEFORE LIGHTS OUT:** Alcohol initially makes you drowsy, but according to the American Academy of Sleep Medicine it keeps you in the lightest stages of sleep, which prevents you from getting the restorative benefits from the other phases. It takes 2 to 3 hours to remove the amount of alcohol from one drink out of your system.

8. **HAVE A NAP STRATEGY:** Daytime snoozes can help you catch up on sleep lost the previous night. The trick is to keep them under 30 minutes—any longer and you may wake up groggy. If you nap regularly, Winter suggests setting a routine nap time so your body clock will expect it.

9. **CHECK YOUR MEDS:** Some medications, including certain antidepressants, beta-blockers, and nonsteroidal anti-inflammatories, such as ibuprofen, can lower melatonin levels. Ask your doc when to take them so they don't interfere with your sleep.

Overtraining

You've heard of overtraining—it's something that happens to elite cyclists who hammer out 600-mile weeks, race in cold rain over nasty cobblestones, and then cap it off with the Tour de France. How could it happen to us mortals when we're lucky to get in 5 or 6 hours a week on the bike, sandwiched by job and family? Falling victim to the big "O" is easier than you think. According to Boston-based triathlon coach Jesse Kropelnicki, owner of QT2 Systems, it's the total stress load in your life that counts—not just the time on the bike. As far as your body is concerned, training is just another stress. Pros routinely ride 20 to 25 hours a week—but that's all they do. Life's little details are handled by team management. (Wouldn't it be nice?) Now look at your schedule. If you're like most people, you're working 40 or more hours per week, shopping, riding, herding kids, juggling a budget, mowing the lawn, and trying to eke out some fitness on the bike. "If you work full time,

10 hours of training each week is a lot," says 1984 Olympic gold medalist Connie Carpenter-Phinney.

SIGNS THAT YOU'RE SINKING

More than 100 symptoms of overtraining have been documented; symptoms range from obvious ones, such as prolonged recovery, to exotica, such as elevated cortisol levels. You should focus on the following five danger signs:

A RACING HEART RATE. Increased resting heart rate is the standard marker of overtraining. Morning heart rate can increase as much as 10 to 15 beats per minute over normal when you're overdoing it. Paradoxically, overtrained cyclists can't get their heart rates as high as usual during hard efforts. This narrowing of the gap between resting and exercise heart rates may be the most telling symptom that you're cooked. You're going slower. More training makes you faster, but only to a point. When your body is overwhelmed by the workload, you'll actually get weaker. In a study of cyclists doing hard intervals two or three times per day for 2 weeks, max power output and time trial times deteriorated quickly.

"HONEY, NOT TONIGHT." Chronic fatigue is often accompanied by depression and apathy. If you used to get fired up just thinking about riding but now can't drag yourself off the couch, you've probably overtrained.

NAGGING AILMENTS. If you get successive colds, suspect overtraining. Studies have shown that the immune system is compromised during periods of high stress, and upper respiratory infections are often the result.

MINOR WOUNDS DON'T HEAL. If you crash and a month later your wounds are still oozing, back off until your body can heal itself.

GROUCHINESS. If you begin to stomp the ground, yell at your significant other, or shriek at drivers, suspect overtraining. Park the bike until you return to your sweet self.

Coming Back from the Dead

So you've been feeling lousy and exhibit the symptoms described here. What's the remedy? There's only one, and you won't like it: rest. Abusing your body got you in this fix, and only some physical and mental time off will set things right. Hang up the bike for a week or more. When you resume riding, cut your usual volume and intensity by half for at least another week. Then increase your distance or pace by no more than 10 percent per week. See if you can reduce stress from other sources in your life. (We know, easier said than done.)

WHEN STOP DOESN'T MEAN GO

You don't wake up one morning to find yourself overtrained—it happens gradually. If you experience one of the six signs below, it's time to start backing off. We show you how.

IF: Your heart rate is higher than normal when you wake up.
THEN: Take an easy or rest day.

IF: You can't stomach the idea of riding.
THEN: Do something else, like a walk or a mellow run or easy swim.

IF: Your heart rate on the bike is unusually high, or it's low plus you're irritable or don't feel well.
THEN: Decrease intensity and/or duration. (Lower heart rate can also signal improved fitness. Keep a training log to become familiar with your body's normal responses.)

IF: You immediately feel horrendous on the bike and have a hard workout planned.
THEN: Spin easy or don't ride.

IF: You feel so-so on the bike and have a hard workout planned.
THEN: Do the first hard effort. If you still don't feel well, spin easy or call it a day.

IF: You didn't sleep well the previous night and don't feel rested.
THEN: Take an easy day.

Compression: Helpful or Hype?

If you've raced a bike in the past few years, you've probably seen that guy—the guy with the tights—out in the parking lot. He wore the tights in the car on the way to the race and maybe slept in them last night. As soon as the race is over, he'll pull his bibs off and roll the squeezing fabrics back on. Maybe it's knee-highs instead of tights. Either way, he'll keep that look for hours, from the postrace diner stop right up until he showers as he seeks to recover from the hard efforts of the day. When it comes to compression, he's a true believer. His legs were fresher than anyone else's, and he's recovering faster. Or so he thinks.

What he's really getting is a little harder to define.

For years, doctors have relied on compression stockings to improve circulation in diabetic and bed-bound patients, as well as to treat lymphedema and phlebitis, among other conditions. The idea is fairly simple: Increased pressure on muscles accelerates the flow of blood to the heart by accentuating human physiology. Blood is pumped to the extremities via high-pressure arteries, but it trickles through low-pressure veins located just beneath the skin on its way back. With added pressure, the blood in those latter veins speeds up. Some time in the 1980s, professional athletes got to thinking: If increased blood flow was good for patients with circulation-related maladies, wouldn't it also benefit them? Soon racers started regularly slipping out of their newfangled spandex shorts (this was the 1980s) and into women's support hose after races.

Thirty years later, compression garments have become a part of our sport and are popular among runners, triathletes, and other athletes. Some of the greatest benefits are claimed by pro cyclists who often face demanding travel schedules: "I wear compression gear almost every waking hour, except for when I'm on the bike," says American pro Craig Lewis.

Compression garment manufacturers claim that wearing their tights and socks can improve recovery speed and, if worn during sports, can boost overall performance. Pros such as Lewis say that they can feel the difference. Ever-increasing numbers of amateur racers—presumably without professional-level travel demands—emulate their heroes by wearing compression garments to the bike shop as well as the race venue. But the question remains: Do athletes get the same benefits from tights as bed-bound patients?

There's minimal evidence to demonstrate

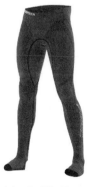

Compression tights feel like the world's best hug.

that compression garments have an impact on recovery for cyclists, despite data showing that they can provide real benefits to runners, says Rob Duffield, PhD, an exercise physiologist at Charles Sturt University in Australia. He has published three compression studies and performed several more for companies that manufacture compression gear. None of his research—or studies performed by others, he says—has convinced him that tight hosiery makes cyclists faster or stronger.

That hasn't stopped some riders from using compression wear, mainly out of a sense that they have nothing to lose. Jeremiah Peiffer, PhD, a competitive cyclist and exercise physiologist at Murdoch University in Australia, regularly wears the garments because he believes in what he calls a "very sound" theory that increased blood flow will lead to better performance and recovery, even as he admits to doubting the benefits are significant. "It's very hard to find a study that makes a clear claim," he says.

The manner in which a human body propels a bike accounts, at least partially, for why compression may not be effective for cyclists. Pedaling is a concentric motion, which means muscles shorten during exertion. In other types of exercise, including running and plyometrics, muscles lengthen as they activate (an eccentric motion). This can lead to delayed-onset muscle soreness, a condition that com-

pression garments can help alleviate during recovery. "It's highly unlikely that you'll get delayed-onset muscle soreness as a cyclist," explains Peiffer, who says that studies performed with runners and other exercisers who use eccentric motion have little relevance for cyclists.

SO WHY DO WE USE THEM?

Every rule has exceptions and, even if most studies have failed to identify a direct benefit, some researchers have reached different conclusions. A 2008 study published in the *International Journal of Sports Physiology and Performance* noted that muscles shrouded in compression garments performed ably on less oxygen. In another study conducted by Matt Driller, PhD, senior researcher at the University of Waikato in New Zealand, the effect of compression garments on back-to-back, 15-minute cycling trials were measured. The study found that cyclists were better able to overcome fatigue and repeat an athletic performance after wearing compression tights.

Triathletes (who obviously also run) are often seen racing in compression gear, but current Union Cycliste Internationale regulations and unwritten (but influential) style rules keep road racers and those who emulate them from wearing compression gear during rides. Still, many cyclists still use them for recovery, claiming benefits above and beyond

RECIPE FOR RECOVERY

THIS POSTWORKOUT RECOVERY DRINK DEVELOPED BY COACH Rick Crawford, a former pro cyclist and triathlete, will help you maximize glycogen replenishment and get ready to hammer the next ride even harder. "Eating normally will provide calories and glycogen, but it may not replace all the glycogen expended," says Crawford, who's coached some of the best cyclists America has produced, including Levi Leipheimer and Tom Danielson. The concoction maximizes your recovery because it combines an easily absorbed food with the muscles' post-ride thirst for glycogen.

Deploy this high-calorie ammunition at the end of a 2-hour (or longer) ride or after a particularly intense effort. Drink it within an hour of your ride, when your muscles are at the peak of receptivity.

RECOVERY BOMB

- 25 grams whey protein isolate (the kind in most high-quality protein powders)

- 70 to 100 grams complex carbohydrate* (1.2 grams per kilogram of body weight)

- 8 ounces grape juice or other sugary liquid

- 1 banana

- 1 cup frozen fruit (Crawford's favorite is blueberries, but mangoes are a close second)

- 8 ounces water

Process all ingredients in a blender until smooth.

MAKES 3 CUPS, OR 1 SERVING

*Look for a pure maltodextrin powder at your local health food store. It gives the best results and the best value. Use a commercial recovery drink in a pinch.

those researchers can identify. Remember, science also cannot fully explain how bicycles are able to remain upright.

IT'S ALL IN OUR HEADS

It's also possible that compression's real benefit—that cyclists say they feel better after using the garments—can be attributed to the placebo effect, in which people imagine benefits that don't have a physical basis. "There may be a perceptual benefit," Duffield notes. "Athletes race how they feel."

If that's the case, then compression has real value, even if it's purely mental. "Athletes believe in [compression garments], and they like them, so there's a benefit for them," says Duffield. If you're an athlete—cyclist, runner, or triathlete—looking for a psychological boost, they may be worth trying, especially if you frequently travel to races or often tackle back-to-back days of big mileage. Before purchasing your own compression clothes, consider the science as well as the anecdotal evidence. You may also consider the distinctive look of compression garments. If you can stomach wearing tights to your bike shop, around your house, and maybe even in public, it may be worth trying them and deciding for yourself if there are benefits. Just don't expect miracles.

CHAPTER 16

Pain Management

People who accumulate lots of road rash over a lifetime have spent their lives happy.

—TIM PARKER, MOUNTAIN BIKER

IN THE BEST OF ALL WORLDS, THE REWARDS OF CYCLING would come without risks. Unfortunately, the sport is a demanding one, and even the most health- and safety-conscious riders are bound to sustain bumps and bruises along the way. Some injuries are self-inflicted: You routinely skip the chamois cream or take a corner too wide. Others, like knee pain, creep up over time. Regardless of whether you're trying to stay healthy or help your body heal, both demand proficiency in one thing: knowing how to listen to your body.

The following chapter covers a variety of physical problems that cyclists face—from wrist pain to saddle sores to broken collarbones. Although you may not need the information now, read it anyhow. Being knowledgeable about possible injuries can help you detect them earlier. And the earlier they're detected, the sooner they can be treated. The sooner they're treated, the faster you can get back on the bike, which is what this is all about anyway, isn't it?

Infamous Annoyances

Our beautiful sport can occasionally give rise to ugly sores, festering boils, and assorted creepy-crawlies. Here's how to avoid a horror show.

CORNEAL ABRASION

Gravel (or was it a bug?) hurtled toward your face and snuck underneath your eyelid, scratching your cornea, the clear, protective covering on your eye.

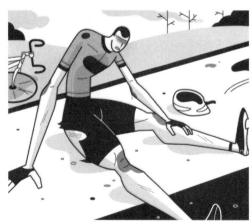

Post-crash, don't rush to stand up. Give your body and your helmet a quick scan.

GET RID OF IT: Listen to your mother: Don't rub your eye. If blinking doesn't work out the debris, flush your eye with clean water or saline solution to prevent further damage. Most minor abrasions will heal without special treatment within a few days. During this time, don't wear contact lenses. More severe eye injuries may require antibiotic drops and a menacing-looking patch from your doctor.

DON'T LET IT HAPPEN AGAIN: Wear protective eyewear to keep out debris. Next time, immediately flush the eye and, again, listen to your mother.

SADDLE SORES

Your saddle, shorts, and the dried salt crystals from sweat can work together like a belt sander on your butt while you pedal. Saddle sores first appear as a mild skin irritation but progress to inflamed hair follicles. Left untreated, they can mutate into infected boils and oozing abscesses.

GET RID OF IT: Take a few days off the bike and keep the affected area clean and dry. Diaper rash and antibiotic creams can soothe the pain and speed up healing. Infected sores require a trip to the doctor and prescription antibiotics, says Gloria Cohen, MD, former physician for the Canadian national and Olympic cycling teams.

DON'T LET IT HAPPEN AGAIN: Adjust your saddle height to reduce chafing and side-to-side hip rocking. Invest in shorts with a seamless chamois, wash them between rides, and use chamois cream.

ROAD RASH

These patches of abraded skin are the result of crashing and sliding across pavement. They are painful but rarely serious, long-lasting, or likely to horrifically scar if treated appropriately.

GET RID OF IT: Quickly get to a place where you can thoroughly clean and disinfect the wound. It is less painful if done within 30 minutes of the crash, because nerve endings are still numb from the trauma. To prevent infection and scarring, scrub the wound hard with a rough washcloth or a medium- or soft-bristle brush. Apply a liberal amount of an antibacterial surgical cleaner, pat the wound dry, then apply an antibacterial ointment (these products are all available without a prescription). Cover the cleaned abrasion with a nonstick sterile dressing. To prevent leakage on clothes or sheets, cover the dressing with a layer of absorbent gauze for the first few days. Change the dressing each morning and night. Apply more antibacterial ointment before covering the wound, and check for signs of infection, such as tenderness, swollen red skin, or a sensation of heat. If you detect any of these, consult a doctor. To minimize scarring, keep the wound moist so a hard scab can't develop. As new skin starts to form, apply a zinc oxide–based salve and light gauze. This kind of salve prevents scabbing. Then use a moisturizer on new skin for at least a week.

DON'T LET IT HAPPEN AGAIN: Avoid crashing. Although that's easier said than done, you can learn to avoid or at least outmaneuver some of the most common causes. See the "Crash Course" section in Chapter 7.

INFECTED ROAD RASH

After that incident involving your shoulder and the road's shoulder, you applied antibacterial ointment for a day, then stopped treating the wound. Unfortunately, it's now a red-hot mess. Literally.

GET RID OF IT: If you remain vigilant, most road rash can be treated with triple-antibiotic ointments. Get to a doctor right away if the road rash feels like a deep bruise, the area is stiff or hard, red streaks radiate from the abrasion, or you have a fever or nausea. Cohen says these symptoms may be signs of compartment syndrome, which can cause long-term muscle and nerve damage, or cellulitis, a spreading infection.

DON'T LET IT HAPPEN AGAIN: Use sterile tweezers or gauze to remove dirt and rocks and sterile water to flush abrasions. Apply antibiotic ointment and bandage the area lightly with a nonstick dressing. Keep the area bandaged for 5 to 6 days. Consistently apply ointments: three times per day or until a dry scab appears, says Cohen.

INGROWN HAIR

The sharp tips of freshly shaved (or improperly waxed) hair can twist and grow back into your skin, especially if you have curly hair.

GET RID OF IT: A warm, wet compress will help soften skin, allowing the hair to grow out. Use tweezers or slip a needle under each hair to gently pull it free. Witch hazel or hydrocortisone cream will help reduce inflammation.

DON'T LET IT HAPPEN AGAIN: Ladies' razor ads model bad shaving behavior. Shave down, not up, going with the grain rather than against it. Soak in hot water and exfoliate your skin before shaving. If you believe extrasmooth skin can trim even more seconds off your time, make a second pass with the razor going left to right, across the grain.

BLACK MOLD

That slime in your water bottle or hydration pack mouthpiece is likely just pesky (and usu- ally harmless) blue-green algae, but it could be harmful bacteria or fungi, such as *Stachybotrys chartarum* (aka black mold), which can cause chronic fatigue, headaches, or worse.

GET RID OF IT: Use a bottle brush or wire tube brush to dislodge the gunk. Then soak the bottle in a 1:10 bleach solution for 10 minutes, says Jon Stabile, owner and chief mechanic of Boulder Bikesmith in Boulder, Colorado. A second soak in water with baking soda should help undo the funky taste.

DON'T LET IT HAPPEN AGAIN: Make a habit of finishing your water by the end of each ride. Then use dish soap and warm water to keep the creepy-crawlies at bay.

CHAFING

It's normal for your butt to feel tender after you return from a long off-season or make a big jump in miles. There's a difference between that type of soreness, which lessens as you adapt, and chafing, where the skin on

SWEET TWEET

THE ONLY THING WORSE THAN ROAD RASH is waking up with the road rash on your legs and ass stuck to your sheets in the middle of the night.

—FORMER CYCLOCROSS NATIONAL CHAMPION RYAN TREBON (@RYANTREBON)

Follow @BicyclingMag on Twitter.

GET FIT

IF YOU'RE SURE YOUR SADDLE IS SET properly and you still have problems, get fit by an expert. Many manufacturers, like Specialized, now offer measurement tools to their dealers. Specialized's Body Geometry Saddle Fit System uses a cushiony seat that retains an imprint of your butt after you sit in it; the dealer's fit expert measures the imprint to find your suggested saddle width, which can solve lingering issues with comfort.

your butt or inner thighs is rubbed raw. Friction causes chafing, which can lead to saddle sores.

GET RID OF IT: If you develop raw spots, clean them gently but well, then slather on an ointment, balm, or diaper rash cream. Don't continue to mask the problem, however. Troubleshoot to find the cause of the chafing: your hips are rocking, your thighs are rubbing the nose of the saddle, and so on.

DON'T LET IT HAPPEN AGAIN: First, always clean down under before and after rides, wear clean shorts, and use chamois cream. If that doesn't help, consider changing your bike seat. A heavily padded saddle sounds like a good solution, but it can actually exacerbate painful saddle issues. As your weight sinks into the saddle, the padding can press into your sensitive nooks, adding pressure where you don't want it. Lightly cushioned seats can be better, especially for longer rides. Persis-

tent issues? See the sidebar "Get Fit." The perfect saddle position puts a platform precisely under your sit bones without pushing you forward, back, or to the side. To hit the spot: Level your saddle and center the rails in the seatpost clamp. Position your seatpost so there's only a slight bend in your knee at the bottom of the pedal stroke. Place the bike on a trainer (level the front with the rear), then have a friend stand behind you to watch your hips as you pedal. If they rock, lower your seatpost slightly. Stop with your cranks at the 3 and 9 o'clock positions and have your friend hold a plumb line against the indentation below your kneecap; the free end of the plumb line should bisect the pedal axle. If it doesn't, move your seat forward or back until it lines up. Avoid messing with saddle tilt. A nose that's too far down will force weight onto your arms; too far back will put pressure in places you don't want to feel it.

Aches and Pains

UPPER BODY

Neck and shoulders cramping up? If it happens early in your ride, you have a fit problem and should visit your local shop for help. If it happens later in your ride, it's likely a tension issue: You're keeping a death grip on the bar or you're simply staying in one position for so long that your muscles are staging a revolt.

"When you're in the same basic position for 1, 2, 3 hours, problems can really come out," says Patrick McCrann, an 18-time Ironman triathlon finisher and author of *Train to Live, Live to Train*. "Taking a few seconds to move around and stretch out can make a big difference."

To help you stay pain free, McCrann suggests the following: a simple exercise to boost your strength and an on-bike stretch to eliminate tension before it becomes full-blown pain.

OFF THE BIKE: Build shoulder and upper-back strength by doing shrugs. Stand with your back straight, legs shoulder-width apart, arms straight at your sides. Hold a relatively light dumbbell in each hand. Breathe out as you pull your shoulders up toward your ears; hold for 1 second, then release. Repeat 6 to 12 times. Do two sets, two or three times a week.

A LITTLE INFLAMMATION GOES A LONG WAY

MOST OF US HEED OUR DOCTOR'S ADVICE to use rest, ice, compression, and elevation to reduce inflammation and speed recovery. Should we also rely on anti-inflammatory measures, such as cortisone injections, large doses of ibuprofen, and other nonsteroidal anti-inflammatory drugs? In a 2010 study done at the Cleveland Clinic in Ohio, researchers concluded that these measures may actually slow healing and that moderation is key. They observed that in acute muscle injuries, inflammatory cells (called macrophages) aided growth that sped muscle regeneration. In other words, a little inflammation actually facilitates healing. This makes anti-inflammatory foods, such as fish and berries, particularly valuable to cyclists on the mend. "These foods throw a big bucket of water on inflammation, but they don't put the fire out entirely," says dietitian Cynthia Sass, MPH, RD.

ON THE BIKE: Sit up and ride with your hands on the top of the handlebar. Move your right hand off the bar and down to your side, palm down. Straighten your arm. Drop your right shoulder slightly as you push your palm toward the pavement; lean your head to the left. You'll feel a stretch in your right neck and shoulder. Hold for a few seconds, relax, switch sides, and repeat as necessary.

KNEES

There's a laundry list of things that can cause knee pain, so let's start with the most common among cyclists: improper leg extension. Your saddle height is either too high or too low. If the pain is in the front of your knee, raise your saddle in 2-millimeter increments until the knee stops complaining. If the pain is in the back, lower your seat instead.

If the pain is under your kneecap, you may have chondromalacia, a softening of the articular cartilage. Muscle imbalances that pull the kneecap out of proper alignment are the most common cause. The repetitive motion of pedaling then irritates and—when left untreated—erodes or shreds the cartilage underneath your kneecap. When this happens, limit your activity, stretch out your legs (extended periods of bent-knee sitting can cause pain), and use ice and anti-inflammatory medicines, such as ibuprofen, to reduce swelling and pain. When you do get back on the bike, stick to the flats and

spin higher cadences and easier gears than usual until the knee is fully healed. To prevent future flare-ups, strengthen your quads and hamstrings: Simple leg extensions in the gym, limiting your range of motion between 30 and 60 degrees, should do the trick. Cleat-position adjustments, a raised saddle, and shorter cranks may help alleviate lateral knee movement, another common contributing factor.

If knee pain persists, or if you just want to prevent injury, there's another action you can take on your own: stretching. The muscles and various connections between your hip and knee can all play a role in knee pain, according to Jeff Guerra, a physical therapist in Boulder, Colorado. "It all acts as one unit," he says. This pigeon stretch works the most overlooked muscles of that unit. Of course, if the pain just won't go away, seek professional help.

THE STANDING PIGEON: Stand in front of a waist-high table or desk. Place your left leg on the table with your knee bent so that your lower leg, from knee to foot, is parallel with the edge of the table. Keeping your hips square and your back flat, bend forward from your hips, not your waist. If this is done correctly, you'll feel the stretch in your hips; incorrectly, you'll feel it in your lower back. To increase the stretch slightly, stand farther away from the table. Hold for 30 seconds to a minute and switch sides. Stretch as often as you like.

ÜBER-FLEXIBLE OPTION: Do the pigeon

stretch on the floor, with your right leg extended behind you as you slowly drop your hips toward the floor.

FEET

Painful burning on the ball of the foot (aka "hot foot," or metatarsalgia) is usually a result of hot weather or poorly fitting shoes—or both—on long, hilly rides. "Pressure can pinch nerves in one or both feet and shut down a ride fast," says Amol Saxena, DPM, a time trial cyclist and podiatrist in the department of sports medicine at the Palo Alto Medical Hospital in California. "If hot foot strikes while you're on a ride, there isn't much you can do other than stop, take off your shoes, and let your feet cool down."

DO THE SQUISH TEST. When shopping for cycling shoes, pull out the insole and hold it up to the bottom of your bare foot (in front of a mirror). "If you can see any part of your foot beyond the borders of the insole, you need a wider shoe," says Saxena.

TAKE A LOAD OFF. Move your cleats a few millimeters closer to the heel of the shoe to take pressure off your forefoot. Or switch to a pedal with a larger platform to more evenly distribute the pressure across your feet.

CUSHION THE BLOW. Over time and after many miles on the bike, your feet start to lose their natural padding, which can make riding painful. Adding more supportive insoles to your cycling shoes can help. If you're shopping for new shoes, take the insoles along to make sure you get the best fit.

BE A MATERIAL GIRL. Choose socks made of high-tech fibers that wick away sweat. Don't buy a pair right off the rack; try them on with your cycling shoes first.

HANDS

About one-quarter of all riders will develop cyclist's palsy, according to Andrew Pruitt, EdD, founder of the Boulder Center for Sports Medicine in Colorado. Symptoms include pain, tingling, numbness, and weakness in the hands, wrists, or fingers.

The culprit is compression of the ulnar nerve, which runs through the wrist and controls sensation in the ring and pinkie fingers as well as motor function in the hand. The solution is taking the pressure off that nerve through proper bike fit and hand positioning. Sitting too far forward or reaching too far to the bar can place undue pressure on your palms. To avoid overextending your wrists, move your hand position often while maintaining neutral or straight wrists. If you're prone to pins and needles, some experts advise stretching and strengthening your lower arms to increase your tolerance for long hours on the bar.

WRIST CURLS: In a seated position, hold a 2-pound dumbbell in one hand and rest your arm on your thigh, with your wrist slightly over your knee, palm up. Let your wrist bend back naturally. Curl the weight up toward your body as far as it will go. Return to start. Do 8 to 10 reps. Then flip your arm so your palm is facing down and complete another set in this position. Switch arms.

WRIST STRETCH: Hold one arm straight, palm down. Drop your fingers toward the floor. With your other hand, gently push on the back of your flexed hand to assist the stretch. Hold 20 seconds. Then extend the hand, pointing your fingertips toward the ceiling. With the opposite hand, gently pull back on your fingers to assist the stretch. Hold 20 seconds. Repeat with opposite hand.

Pro Tip

Occasionally take one hand off the bar and shake it. This relaxes your shoulder and elbow and encourages blood flow to your hand to prevent numbness.

The Pain Game

Some athletes try to block pain before it starts by taking ibuprofen or other nonsteroidal anti-inflammatory drugs before a tough workout or race. According to a study by researchers at Appalachian State University and Vanderbilt University published in *Medicine and Science in Sports and Exercise*, this practice may be

unhealthy in the long-term. Extreme marathon runners took 600 milligrams of ibuprofen before a race and experienced significantly higher levels of oxidative stress than racers who took nothing. Oxidative stress causes increased production of cell-damaging free radicals and has been linked to certain cancers, faster aging, and Alzheimer disease. Popping a few ibuprofen before a century will prevent pain, but in the long run you might be better off toughing it out.

After intense rides or even injuries, if you want to feel better faster, try adding foods and drinks to your diet that act like natural ibuprofen, says Mary Miles, PhD, associate professor of movement science and nutrition at Montana State University in Bozeman. Unlike man-made anti-inflammatory agents, says Miles, "they have antioxidant properties that may decrease muscle damage, speed recovery, and possibly enhance performance."

BLACK OR GREEN TEA: Sports scientists at Rutgers University found that a 9-day supplement of black tea extract decreased delayed-onset muscle soreness after cycling intervals. "The black tea extract reduces the oxidative stress of the exercises and speeds recovery between intervals," says Shawn Arent, PhD, assistant professor at Rutgers University in New Brunswick, New Jersey.

TO RECHARGE: "Add four bags of decaffeinated tea to 32 ounces of cold water and steep in the refrigerator overnight," suggests

Barbara Lewin, RD, a sports nutritionist who owns Sports-Nutritionist.com. Drink tea in place of water before, during, and after rides.

SOYBEANS AND TOFU: The branched-chain amino acids in soybeans stop muscle degradation during long rides, and the antioxidants found in soy help alleviate post-ride aches and pains. Research published in *The Nutrition Journal* found that both soy and whey proteins build lean muscle mass, but soy protein also prevents exercise-induced inflammation.

TO RECHARGE: "Chocolate soy milk makes an excellent recovery drink," says Lewin. Also, keep soy nuts in the car or at the office for a great protein-rich snack.

SALMON AND TUNA: Though we don't usually think of fatty foods as performance-enhancers, the omega-3 fatty acids in salmon and tuna go way beyond serving as an energy source. "Omega-3s generally increase blood flow," says Jay Udani, MD, medical director of the integrative medicine program at the David Geffen School of Medicine at the University of California, Los Angeles. "This may help wash out inflammatory cells in damaged muscles" that cause pain and swelling.

TO RECHARGE: Keep canned salmon and tuna on hand for sandwiches and salads. Aim for two to three servings a week.

TURMERIC: Loaded with a potent anti-inflammatory compound called curcumin, this yellow spice may help to increase endurance and speed recovery. In a 2007 study at the University of South Carolina, exercise physiologists gave mice curcumin supplements for 3 days before a 2.5-hour downhill run. The curcumin reduced muscle inflammation and increased endurance by more than 20 percent the next day.

TO RECHARGE: Make turmeric your go-to spice. Add it to marinades, rice, vegetables, and so on. You'll hardly notice the subtle flavor.

CHERRIES AND BERRIES: In a study at the University of Vermont, students who were given 12 ounces of tart cherry juice before and after strenuous exercises suffered only a 4 percent reduction in muscle strength the next day compared with a 22 percent loss found in subjects given a placebo. "Antioxidants and anti-inflammatory molecules in tart cherries suppress and treat the microtears in muscles," says Declan Connolly, PhD. These molecules are also found in blackberries, raspberries, and strawberries.

TO RECHARGE: Stock up on frozen berries and add them to smoothies, yogurt, and cereal. Or defrost a few in the microwave for a sweet post-ride snack.

CRAMPING

When it comes to curing muscle cramps, there's no shortage of folk wisdom remedies. Popular "solutions" include drinking water, eating bananas, stretching, doing plyometrics, or just plain slowing down. Of course, you could try taking calcium, salt, magnesium, or quinine (a drug for malaria). Hey, why not? It's been tried before.

The truth is that although scientists have studied cramps for more than 50 years, we still don't understand the cause. We do know that some people are inexplicably prone to getting them, while others are perennially cramp free; cramps are more common during competition, so overexertion seems to be a factor; they're common in the hours after prolonged exercise; and nutrition can play a role for some people.

Unfortunately, there's little scientific evidence that inadequate fluid or sodium intake causes cramps. In one study, 15 runners who developed cramps during a marathon were compared to 67 who didn't. There were no differences in hydration or sodium levels between the two groups. What's more, dehydration doesn't explain the cramps that occur several hours after riding, when hydration has been restored.

Magnesium plays a role in muscle contraction, and a shortage of this mineral can result in severe muscle cramping; however, low blood levels of magnesium are rare. In a study of Hawaii Ironman triathletes with cramps, adding magnesium to intravenous fluids didn't help. Although eating bananas, a source of potassium, is often cited as a remedy for cramps, there's little evidence it helps. Potas-

sium deficiency results from using some diuretics, prolonged vomiting, chronic diarrhea, or laxative abuse, not from sweating.

With no scientific agreement on how to prevent cramps, what's a cyclist to do?

KEEP DRINKING. Hydration seems to work for some people, even if there is no direct scientific link between it and cramp prevention. It's still critical to all other aspects of performance, so drink up.

BOOST SODIUM INTAKE. This is especially important if you perspire heavily. Daily sweat losses of 4 to 6 pounds or more could lead to a sodium deficit in someone on a low-sodium diet, possibly contributing to cramping. Each pound of sweat contains 200 to 400 milligrams of sodium, and a diet with few processed or salty foods could contain less than 2,000 milligrams of sodium daily. Try adding 1,500 to 2,000 milligrams more sodium to your usual daily diet for 2 weeks to see if it helps. Most North Americans get more than enough salt in their diets, although sweating cyclists may be an exception. The concentration of sodium in sweat varies so widely that exact guidelines are impossible to suggest. (Don't worry about elevating your blood pressure, as increasing your sodium intake moderately for a 2-week trial period won't affect blood pressure over the long term.) If you haven't noticed fewer cramps in 2 weeks, low sodium obviously wasn't a factor and you should return to your normal intake.

STRETCH. Calf cramps can often be relieved while riding by standing on the bike and dropping the heel at the bottom of the pedal stroke. For cramps in the front of the thigh, unclip your foot and raise it toward your buttocks. Stretch your quads by gently pulling on the foot with the same-side hand. (Be careful: In some cases, this may lead to cramps in your hamstrings!) Stretching also works to relieve cramps that occur after riding.

RIDE WITHIN YOUR LIMITS. Overexertion seems to cause some cramps, so don't jump into rides that are too hard for your current training. A good rule: Don't increase mileage more than 10 percent a week.

HAMSTRING STRAIN

Cyclists often come to Anna Saltonstall, a physical therapist at Mid-Columbia Medical Center in The Dalles, Oregon, with hamstring strains that could have been prevented. Improper bike fit is one of the leading causes of the injury, according to Saltonstall. "If your seat is too far back, you overuse your hamstrings and glutes, and if it's too high, you overextend your hamstrings with each pedal stroke," she says. "Saddles that put too much pressure on the sciatic nerve, which feeds the hamstrings, can cause numbness and pain in those muscles."

Even on properly fitted bikes, cyclists stress their hamstrings when climbing hills, espe-cially when seated and using a high gear. Stronger hamstrings are less prone to injury, so Saltonstall suggests incorporating resistance training into days spent off the bike. Also, she recommends preceding each ride with a warm-up that lasts at least 5 minutes, followed by thorough stretching of potential problem areas.

TO STRENGTHEN: Lie on your back, knees bent, feet directly under knees. With shoulder blades and head on the floor, raise your butt to align with your thighs. Hold for 30 seconds. Complete five repetitions.

ACHILLES TENDINITIS

Feel a twinge near the bottom of your calf or the back of your ankle when you're sprinting, grunting up a long climb, or pushing a big gear? It could be that your Achilles tendon is inflamed, a common occurrence caused by microtears in the tendon, often caused by overuse. Continue to push through the pain, and tendinitis could force you out of the saddle for 4 to 6 weeks. Or pay attention to your Achilles now to prevent problems later.

To do that, first try raising the saddle and going for an easy spin while pedaling lightly, then see if the discomfort lessens. Increasing the distance from the saddle to the pedal seems to defy logic, but sometimes when the saddle is low, a cyclist's foot is in such a horizontal position, with the ankle bent at a right angle, that it causes strain on the tendon. Raising the saddle results in the foot being pointed slightly downward. Next, stretch. "Stretching on a regular basis is enormously helpful because the increased pliability can prevent microtearing," says Fiona Lockhart, USA Cycling expert coach. "Plus, stretching improves blood flow to the area, which speeds healing."

Work these simple stretches into your daily routine, and you'll keep your Achilles tendon supple, pliable, and ready to turn the cranks at a moment's notice.

THE BASEBOARD BLAST: Remove your shoes and stand facing a wall, slightly less than arm's length away. Press the ball of your right foot against the wall with your foot angled up, so that only your heel touches the floor. Your leg should be extended slightly in front of you. Slowly bring your chest toward the wall until you feel a stretch in your calf. Hold for 30 seconds. Repeat with your left leg.

THE STAIR DROP: Stand on the edge of a step and drop your right heel until you feel the stretch. (If it's painful, stop. You're only making the microtear worse.) Hold for 30 seconds. Release. Repeat with left heel. Do periodically throughout the day.

SHOULDER INJURIES

Collarbone fractures and shoulder separations often result from "plop" falls, when you're going slowly, so you put out a hand to catch yourself and the impact is transferred to the shoulder. Faster, sliding falls often spare your shoulder, wrist, and arm (but carry their own delightful consequences).

When you hit the ground, you'll feel pain and maybe hear a popping sound. There may also be visible deformity. With broken collarbones (this injury accounts for 23 percent of all fractures sustained by recreational riders, and 58 percent of all racers' snapped bones) you'll see and feel a bump. Shoulder separations produce pain and swelling of the acromioclavicular joint where the collarbone meets the shoulder blade.

QUICK FIX: There isn't a quick fix for this one. Nine out of 10 collarbone breaks don't require surgery but are fixed by immobilizing the bone with a sling. Riding with a broken collarbone (or acromioclavicular joint separation) is dangerous for bike handling reasons and can complicate the healing process. So relax, rest, and heal.

LONG-TERM CARE: See a physician immediately. You don't have to go to the emergency room. Instead, go directly to an orthopedist. Inquire about stationary training as a means to preserve your hard-won fitness until you can get back on the road or trail.

Concussions

Brain injuries are on the rise. Between 1997 and 2011 the number of bike-related concussions suffered annually by American riders increased by 67 percent, from 9,327 to 15,546, according to the National Electronic Injury Surveillance System, a yearly sampling of hospital emergency rooms conducted by the US Consumer Product Safety Commission.

Of course, concussions are more readily diagnosed now than they were 15 years ago, which likely accounts for some of the increase. It's also possible that increased helmet use has led to more lives saved and thus to more people being lumped into the brain injury category. Still, this doesn't account for thousands of cases. We're left with this stark statistical fact: The concussion rate among bicycle riders has grown faster than the sport.

If you crash and hit your head, there are two types of impact. One is known as linear acceleration. That's the impact of the skull meeting the pavement. Today's helmets do an excellent job of preventing catastrophic injury and death by attenuating that blow.

The second type is known as rotational acceleration. This is where things get tricky. Even if the skull isn't damaged, it still stops short. That causes the brain to rotate (the technical term is *inertial spin*), which creates shear strain. Imagine a plate of fruit gelatin being jarred so hard that little cuts open throughout the jiggly mass. That strain can damage the axons that carry information between neurons within the brain.

There are other factors involved, but

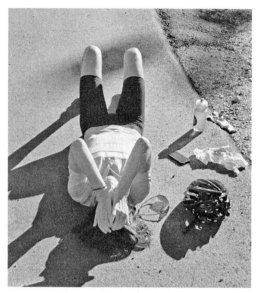

You don't have to lose consciousness to suffer a concussion.

research has consistently pointed to rotational acceleration as the biggest single factor in a concussion's severity. The US Consumer Product Safety Commission helmet benchmark is based solely on linear acceleration. There's never been a standards test, required or voluntary, for rotational acceleration. In other words, bicycle helmets do an outstanding job keeping our skulls intact in a major crash, but they do almost nothing to prevent concussions and other significant brain injuries.

WHAT TO LOOK FOR

Symptoms can span days or weeks. If you experience any of these, see a doctor.

HEADACHE: Ninety-five percent of concussed athletes get them, according to the *American Journal of Sports Medicine.*

WHEN YOU NOTICE IT: Within 30 minutes (severe pain that day; mild afterward)

SENSITIVITY: A concussion can disrupt brain circuits, causing bright lights and noises to seem more intense.

WHEN YOU NOTICE IT: From immediately after the injury up to a few days beyond

NAUSEA SYMPTOMS: Unrelenting or intense nausea or vomiting after a crash may indicate a more severe concussion. Get to an emergency room.

WHEN YOU NOTICE IT: Within the first few hours

DIZZINESS: Concussions can cause bruising or trauma in the inner ear, which can make you feel as if you have been whirling around or have vertigo.

WHEN YOU NOTICE IT: Usually within minutes

MEMORY LOSS: You may forget the crash—or the ambulance ride afterward. This could indicate a particularly severe concussion even if your memory returns within minutes.

WHEN YOU NOTICE IT: Right after the injury

MENTAL FATIGUE: If you daily routine is suddenly exhausting, you're still recovering from the concussion.

WHEN YOU NOTICE IT: The second or third day after the injury

IRRITABILITY: Think mood swings and a short temper that has you lashing out.

WHEN YOU NOTICE IT: A few days later, even after the physical symptoms subside

HOW TRAUMATIC BRAIN INJURY IS TREATED

Doctors recommend that anyone who shows even the slightest symptom of a head injury should seek medical attention. People who are diagnosed with the mildest head injuries may be treated as outpatients or be referred to neuropsychologists, who provide medication and rehabilitation exercises to improve function despite impairments. More severe cases usually warrant immediate hospitalization, where patients may remain for 2 to 3 weeks as their condition is stabilized. For example, a coma may be medically induced to allow the brain time to begin healing and part of the skull may be cut away to reduce swelling.

As the patient regains strength, rehabilitation begins. "Early therapy helps brain cells that are bruised or stunned to recover their function faster," says Darryl Kaelin, MD, medical research director of the Acquired Brain Injury Program at the Shepherd Center in Atlanta. "Later, rehab trains brain cells not involved in a particular activity to pick up for the ones that have been destroyed."

This process can focus on relearning basic functions, such as how to walk, or overcoming some of the more bewildering aspects of head trauma. As the messages of the brain are scrambled or lost by the disconnected axons and other parts of the brain try to compensate, patients may speak gibberish, lash out physically, exhibit wild and childish behavior, or discover they can fluently speak a second language. Repeating simple tasks helps the brain heal and begin properly sending its messages again. This can take months or years.

THE PROGNOSIS

Most people who suffer mild head trauma recover in 6 to 12 months. The outlook for moderate and severe injuries is less hopeful. "Not many people with moderate to severe injuries fully recover, in terms of the brain working exactly like it used to," says Lance Trexler, PhD, director of the department of rehabilitation neuropsychology at the Rehabilitation Hospital of Indiana in Indianapolis. "About 50 percent do not resume their full activities and live with a chronic disability." This can range from keeping a notebook to compensate for memory loss, coping with chronic odd behaviors that arise from the brain's internal misfire, to a vegetative state or coma in severe cases.

Even for the fully recovered patient, the injury remains a significant part of their lives: It increases the chance another knock on the head will prove traumatic. "After one injury your threshold is lower, and a smaller hit can inflict the same damage," says Douglas H. Smith, MD, director of Philadelphia's Penn Center for Brain Injury and Repair. "Mind your brain—don't sacrifice not being you anymore."

Foods That Heal

When an injury sidelines a cyclist, the natural reaction is to cut back on calories until it's time to ride and burn energy again, but the healing process demands fuel, too. "It's like fixing a house," says sports dietitian Cynthia

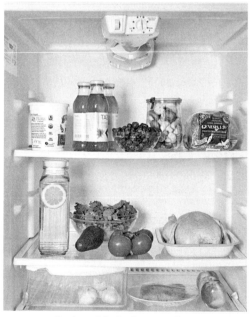

Feed your injuries to recover fast.

Sass, MPH, RD. "A crack in the foundation requires raw materials to patch things back together, and in the body those raw materials come from what we eat." Proteins, vitamins, minerals, and antioxidants help heal wounds, relax stressed tendons, and mend fractured bones more quickly. So in addition to your doctor's advice to elevate and ice, choose the right combinations of foods to speed recovery and get back on your bike. Here's where to aim your cart at the grocery store.

PRODUCE SECTION

BUY: Carrots, spinach, sweet potatoes, and kale for vitamin A; oranges, strawberries, peppers, and broccoli for vitamin C

WHY: Vitamin A helps make white blood cells for fighting infection, "which is always a risk with injury," says Sass. Vitamin C has been proven to help skin and flesh wounds heal faster and stronger, making it a valuable ally when caring for road rash. Vitamin C also helps repair connective tissues and cartilage by contributing to the formation of collagen, an important protein that builds scar tissue, blood vessels, and even new bone cells.

MEAT COUNTER

BUY: Lean turkey, sirloin, fish, and chicken

WHY: Lean meats are packed with protein, a critical building block for producing new cells. In a 2008 study published in the *Journal of the Federation of American Societies for Experimental Biology*, researchers at the University of Ottawa identified a protein that acted like a bridge between damaged tissues, promoting repair. For optimum healing, athletes require about 112 grams of protein per day (for a 175-pound male or female), and eating meat is an easy way to rocket toward this goal faster.

DAIRY DEPARTMENT

BUY: Eggs, milk, and yogurt

WHY: All three are good sources of protein; milk and yogurt also contain calcium, which repairs bone and muscle. The vitamin D in dairy products improves calcium absorption and helps injured muscle and bone heal: A 2010 study published in the *Journal of Bone and Joint Surgery* reported that boosting this nutrient's levels in deficient patients produced earlier results.

CEREAL AISLE

BUY: Fortified cereal

WHY: These cereals contain zinc, a proven asset to the immune system and to healing wounds. Along with red meat, fortified cereals are the best sources (some deliver 100 percent of your recommended daily value). By itself, zinc doesn't repair damaged tissue, but it assists the nutrients that do. "Just don't overdo it," Sass cautions, adding that too much of this potent mineral lowers HDL cholesterol (the good kind) and actually suppresses your immune system. Adults shouldn't exceed 40 grams of zinc a day. Cereal supplies moderate zinc doses as well as whole grain carbohydrates, which fuel your body's healing efforts and keep it from dipping into protein for energy. "Eating enough carbs ensures that your body puts all of its available protein toward repairs," Sass explains.

SEAFOOD CASE

BUY: Salmon, tuna, and trout

WHY: In addition to an added protein bonus, fish is packed with omega-3s, fatty acids that quench the inflammation that slows recovery from tendinitis, bone fractures, and sprained ligaments.

Further Reading

HOPEFULLY THIS BOOK HAS GIVEN YOU EVERYTHING YOU NEED TO KICK-start your training, but as you're about to find out, racing is a life-long learning experience. Most of your education will happen on the bike, but to make the most of your experiences, you have to know what to expect beforehand and how to interpret your results afterward. These books, which include many of my faves, will help you to continue to boost your training and racing IQ—or just fall more in love with the sport—from now until the end of your career. Happy reading.

EVEN MORE TRAINING ADVICE

Get Fast! A Complete Guide to Gaining Speed Wherever You Ride, by Selene Yeager, Rodale 2013

The Cyclist's Training Bible, by Joe Friel, Velo Press 2009

The Time-Crunched Cyclist: Fit, Fast, Powerful in 6 Hours a Week, by Chris Carmichael and Jim Rutberg, Velo Press 2012

CYCLOCROSS

Cyclocross: Training and Technique, by Simon Burney and Richard Fries, Velo Press 2007

Mud, Snow, and Cyclocross: How 'Cross Took Over US Cycling, by Molly Hurford, Deeds Publishing 2012

The Complete Book of Cyclocross, Skill Training, and Racing, by Scott R. Mares, Siberian Express LLC 2008.

MOUNTAIN BIKING

Mastering Mountain Bike Skills, 2nd edition, by Brian Lopes and Lee McCormack, Human Kinetics, 2010

Mountain Bike Like a Champion, by Ned Overend, Ben Hewitt, and Ed Pavelka, Rodale 1999

The Mountain Biker's Training Bible, by Joe Friel, Velo Press 2000

NUTRITION AND HYDRATION

The Feed Zone Cookbook: Fast and Flavorful Food for Athletes, by Biju K. Thomas and Allen Lim, Velo Press 2011

Feed Zone Portables: A Cookbook of On-the-Go Food for Athletes, by Biju K. Thomas, Allen Lim, Taylor Phinney, and Tim Johnson, Velo Press 2013

Racing Weight Cookbook: Lean, Light Recipes for Athletes, by Matt Fitzgerald and Georgie Fear, Velo Press 2014

The Cyclist's Food Guide: Fueling for the Distance, by Nancy Clark, MS, RD, and Jenny Hegmann, MS, RD, Sports Nutrition Publishers 2011.

INSPIRATION

Boy Racer: My Journey to Tour de France Record-Breaker, by Mark Cavendish, Velo Press 2010

Pro Cycling on $10 a Day: From Fat Kid to Euro Pro, by Phil Gaimon, Velo Press 2014

Rusch to Glory: Adventure, Risk & Triumph on the Path Less Traveled, by Rebecca Rusch with Selene Yeager, Velo Press 2014

STRATEGY

Racing Tactics for Cyclists, by Thomas Prehn and Charles Pelkey, Velo Press 2004

Reading the Race: Bike Racing from Inside the Peloton, by Jamie Smith and Chris Horner, Velo Press 2013

STRENGTH TRAINING

Tom Danielson's Core Advantage: Core Strength for Cycling's Winning Edge, by Tom Danielson, Allison Westfahl, and Patrick Dempsey, Velo Press 2013

Foundation: Redefine Your Core, Conquer Back Pain, and Move with Confidence, by Eric Goodman, Peter Park, and Lance Armstrong, Rodale 2011

Weight Training for Cyclists: A Total Body Program for Power & Endurance, by Ken Doyle and Eric Schmitz, Velo Press 2008

TRAINING TOOLS

Bicycling Training Journal: 52 Weeks of Motivation, Training Tips, Cycling Wisdom, and Much More for Every Kind of Cyclist, by the editors of *Bicycling* magazine, Rodale 2012

The Power Meter Handbook: A User's Guide for Cyclists and Triathletes, by Joe Friel, Velo Press 2012

Training and Racing with a Power Meter, by Hunter Allen and Andrew Coggan, Velo Press 2010

WEIGHT LOSS

Bike Your Butt Off! A Breakthrough Plan to Lose Weight and Start Cycling (No Experience Necessary!), by Selene Yeager and Leslie Bonci, Rodale 2014

Racing Weight: How to Get Lean for Peak Performance (The Racing Weight Series), by Matt Fitzgerald, Velo Press 2012

WRENCH WORK

The Bicycling Guide to Complete Bicycle Maintenance & Repair: For Road & Mountain Bikes, by Todd Downs, Rodale 2012

Zinn and the Art of Mountain Bike Maintenance, by Lennard Zinn and Todd Telander, Velo Press 2010

Zinn and the Art of Road Bike Maintenance: The World's Best-Selling Bicycle Repair and Maintenance Guide, by Lennard Zinn, Velo 2013

Acknowledgments

THIS BOOK WOULD NOT HAVE BEEN POSSIBLE WITHOUT *BICYCLING*'S many expert columnists and contributors, especially the following, whose work appears regularly in these pages.

Chris Carmichael is a former Olympic and Tour de France cyclist and the founder of Carmichael Training Systems (trainright.com). He's authored multiple books, including *The Time-Crunched Cyclist*.

James Herrera is an exercise physiologist, researcher, educator, US national team coach, and the founder of Performance Driven Coaching (pushyourlimit.com). Follow him on Twitter: @poweredbyplants.

Joe Friel is an endurance sports coach, cofounder of Training Bible Coaching (trainingbible.com) and TrainingPeaks.com and is the author of *The Cyclist's Training Bible*, among many other books. Follow him on Twitter: @jfriel.

Selene Yeager is a USA Cycling certified coach and elite mountain bike racer. In addition to writing *Bicycling*'s "Fit Chick" column, she's also authored numerous books, including *Bike Your Butt Off!*, *Get Fast!*, and *Ride Your Way Lean*. Follow her on Twitter: @FitChick3.

Photograph and Illustration Credits

Jack Affleck, page 196

Douglas Benedict, page 164

Chris Bersbach, page 139

Beth Bischoff, page 93, 94, 95

Serge Bloch, *page 42*

Gerard Brown, page 128

Levi Brown, page 51

Harry Campbell, *page 238*

Leela Cyd, page 252

Michael Darter, pages 190, 202

Tara Donne, page 92

Jered Gruber, page 151

Haisam Hussein, *page 104*

Getty Images, pages 107, 165, 201

James + Therese, pages 85, 86, 87

Charlie Layton, *pages 68. 69, 70, 71, 73, 74, 75, 76, 77*

Jesse Lenz, page 124

Colby Lysne, page 183

Thomas MacDonald, pages 89, 90, 91

Kagan McLeod, *page 78*

Camille McMillan, page 156

Brakethrough Media, page 4

Barbara Minafra, page 140

Sophie Pangrazzi, page 228

Dan Patitucci, page 109

Francois Portmann, page 101

Michael Robertson, pages 105, 58, 220

Marc Rosenthal, *page 134*

Bob Scott, page 179

Lisa Shin, page 55

Dave Silver, page 194

Angie Smith, page 115

Zoot Sports, page 233

Jake Stangel, page 250

Kyle Webster, pages 84, 85, 86, 87

Stephen Wilde, page 14

Index

Boldface page references indicate photographs. Underscored references indicate boxed text or tables.

A

Abdominal strength training exercise, 80
Acceleration phase of sprint, <u>106</u>, <u>107</u>
Achilles tendinitis, 248–49
Acidosis, 7
Active recovery
  training zone, 30, <u>30</u>
  workouts, 135, <u>135</u>, 143, <u>144–45</u>, 207, <u>208–9</u>
Active rest. *See* Rest
Adaptation, muscular, 226
Adenosine, 60
Aero, 28, 150, 158, 170–72
Aero bars, 171–72
Aerobic capacity, 5–6
Aerobic system, 5–6
Aerodynamics, 28, 150, 158, 170–72
Alcohol, 220–21, 230–31
Allen, Hunter, 15, 213, 216–18, 226
All-in-one tool, 81
Alveoli, 33
American Bicycle Racing, 152
Amino acids, 48, 246
Anaerobic capacity
  power builders workouts, 185, <u>186–87</u>
  training zone, 30–31, <u>30</u>
Anaerobic system, 6–7
Anaerobic threshold. *See* Lactate
  threshold

Anding, Roberta, 47–48
Andreu, Frankie, 114, <u>155</u>
Apex of turn, 102, 117, 193, 197–98, 203
Appetite and sugar, 46
Applegate, Andy, 114–15
Applegate, Liz, 49–50
Arent, Shawn, 245
Arm strength training exercises
  Applause Pushup, 80
  effects of, 77
  Hammer Curl, 78, **78**
  Lying Triceps Extension, 78, **78**
  Military Pushup, 78, **78**
Armstrong, Lance, 63
Arm warmers, removing while riding, 115
Artery health, <u>90</u>
Ascending hills. *See* Climbing
Athlete's Plate, The, 54
Attacking
  in criterium races, 166
  drill, 113
  improving, 113
  in one-day road race, 161
  workouts, 113

B

Back
  foam roller stretching exercise, 94, **94**
  pain management, 88, <u>89</u>

strength training exercise, 80
stretching, 88
Bars, nutritional, 55–57, **55**
Bar tape, cleaning, 179
Base period of macrocycle
  describing, 12–13
  sample year training, 16–17
  strength training during
    arms, 77–78, **78**
    core, 75–76, **75–76**
    glutes, 73–74, **73–74**
    legs, 70–72, **70–72**
Bass, Rich, 3
Bavineau, Marc, 139
Beans, 48
Beef, 49, <u>74</u>
Belly breathing, 34
Berms, handling high-banked, 197–98
Berries, 52–53, 246
Beverages. *See* Drinks; Hydration
Bicycle Racing Association of Colorado, 152
Bicycling.com/eventfinder, 165
Bicycling flexibility test
  calves, 87, **87**
  glutes, 86, **86**
  hamstrings, 87, **87**
  iliotibial band, quads, hip flexors, 84–86, **84–86**

body position, 28, <u>106</u>, 108, 203–4
carrying, 182, **183**, 199
chain, lubricating, 179
cleaning, 178
computer, 19–20
cyclocross, <u>182</u>
falling off, 118–19
fit, 32, 139, 171–72
fork, setting and checking, <u>205</u>
frame, checking after crashing, 120
helmet, 119–20, 250
maintenance, 178–79
mountain, <u>183</u>
preparation, 124, 178–79
rebound of suspension, <u>205</u>
road, <u>182</u>
sag, measuring suspension's, <u>205</u>
shocks, setting and adjusting, <u>205</u>
stationary, 24
tires, inflating, 179
Bike lifts workouts, 185, <u>186–87</u>
Black mold in water bottle, 240
Black tea, 245
Blended periodization, 15–16
Bliss, Karen, 105
Blood lactate level. *See* Lactate threshold
Body composition, 215–17
Body fat, 46, 49
Body position, bike, 18, <u>106</u>, 108, 203–4
Body shape, <u>222</u>
Body weight. *See* Cycling weight; Weight
Bonci, Leslie, <u>53</u>, <u>55</u>, 221–22
Bone density and mass, 32, 54
Borg, Gunnar, 23
Borg scale, 23–25
Brainard, Golden, 190, 195
Brain chemistry, 46, 60
Brain injuries, 249–54
Brake pads, fresh, 101
Brakes, checking after crashing, 120
Braking
    cornering and, 100–102
    drill, 195
    emergency, 100–101
    erratic, avoiding, 102
    finger position and, 100
    in mountain bike races and riding, 195–96
    pressure and, applying evenly, 100
    "right rear" rule and, 100
    skills, tips for, 100–102
Brandt Hauptmann, Laurie, 200
Breakdowns, preparing for bike, 204, <u>205</u>, 206

Breakfast, <u>55</u>, 62–63, 223
Breaking away in race, 161–62
Breathing
    belly, 34
    deep, 35
    lungs and, 33–35
    normal, 33
    Pro Tip, <u>133</u>
    shallow, 33–34
    for stress management, <u>133</u>
    before switchbacks, 202
    synchronizing, 34
    tests, 34
Breus, Michael, 230
Brick workouts, 185, <u>186–87</u>
Brooks, George A., 7
Browning, Julie, <u>166</u>
Build period of macrocycle
    describing, 13
    in sample year training, 17–18
    strength training during, 79–80
Bunny hop move, 184
Bursts workouts, 162, <u>163</u>, 173, <u>174–75</u>, 185, <u>186–87</u>

C

Cadence, 109, <u>125</u>
Caffeine
    absorption of, 61–62, 230
    carbohydrates and, <u>45</u>
    dehydration and, myth of, 61
    in diet, 60–62
    dietary fats and, 60
    endurance and, 60
    facts about, 61–62
    hydration and, 61
    intake of, recommended, 60–61, 230
    muscles and, 60
    performance and, 60–62
    power output and, 60
    side effects of, 61
    sleep and, 230
    sources of, 61
    tolerance to, 61
    use of, common, 60
Calcium, 49, 53–54
California Bicycle Racing, 152
Calories, 220–21
Calves
    bicycling flexibility test, 87, **87**
    foam roller stretching exercise, 95, **95**
    stretching, 87, **87**
Capillaries, 5

Carbohydrates
    absorption of, 43–45
    bars, 56
    for breakfast, 62
    caffeine and, <u>45</u>
    complex, 43
    confusing information about, 42
    in diet, 42–45, 47, <u>47</u>
    in drinks, 45, 58
    endurance and, 42–43
    facts about, 42–45
    intake of, recommended, 45, 47, 47, 66
    loading up on, 62–63
    muscles and, 8
    performance and, 45
    refueling during riding and, 66
    simple, 43
    sources of, 43, 63
    stored, 8
Carbo-loading, 62–63
Carmichael Training field test, **25**
Carpenter-Phinney, Connie, 231
Carrying bike, 182, **183**, 199
Carrying gear and food while riding, 128
Carter, Michael, 164, 166
Carver, Todd, 103–5, 171
Casa, Douglas, 59–60
Casein, 49
"Cat 5 tattoo," avoiding, 156
Century rides
    bike preparation for, 124
    body position changes during, 125
    carrying gear and food while riding in, 128
    diet and, 125–28
    double century rides, 128–29
    gear for, 129
    gran fondos vs., 138, <u>138</u>
    hydration and, 125, 127
    pacing in, 125
    planning for, 124–25
    rest during, 125, 127
    as rite of passage, 123
    tips for, 124–25, <u>125</u>
    training for, <u>126</u>, 128–29, <u>130</u>
    workouts for, 129, <u>130</u>
Cereals, 253–54
Chafing, 240–41
Chain, lubricating bike, 179
Charity Navigator, 132–33
Charity rides
    describing, 132
    fund-raising goal and, 133–34
    pack riding in, <u>134</u>, <u>135</u>
    selecting, 132–33

Charity rides (*cont.*)
    training for, 134–36, <u>135</u>, <u>136–37</u>
    workouts for, 135–36, <u>135</u>, <u>136–37</u>
Cherries, 53, 246
Cheung, Stephen, 225, 227
Chicken, dark meat, 49
Chocolate soy milk, 246
Cholesterol, 50
Chondromalacia, 243
Christen, Carson, 85
Chronic ailments as overtraining
        symptom, 232
Chronic fatigue as overtraining
        symptom, 232
Cinnamon, 52
Clark, Nancy, 229
Cleaning bike, 178
Cleat position, 139
Cleats and foot pain, 244
Climbing
    cadence and, 109
    counting strategy for mental
            toughness and, <u>166</u>
    drill, 113, 191
    hamstring strain and, 248
    improving, 113
    in mountain bike races and riding,
            191–92
    while pack riding, 110
    pedaling and, <u>110</u>
    Pro Tip, <u>110</u>, <u>111</u>
    on rolling terrain, 109
    shifting while, <u>111</u>, 139
    short and steep hills, 110
    skills, tips for, 108–10, **109**, <u>110</u>, <u>111</u>
    workouts, 110–11, 113, 207, <u>208–9</u>
Climb repeats workouts, 207, <u>208–9</u>
Clothing, 140, 233–34, **233**, 236
Coffee, 61. *See also* Caffeine
Coggan, Andrew, 27
Cohen, Gloria, 239
Cold bath and recovery, 228–29, **228**
Collarbone fractures, 249
Competition. *See* Racing; *specific race
        name*
Complex carbohydrates, 43
Compression clothing, 232–34, **233**, 236
Compression, measuring bike
        suspension's, <u>205</u>
Computer, bike and cycling, 19, 20
Concussions, 249–54
Connolly, Declan, 246
Consumer Product Safety Commission,
        250
Contador, Alberto, 116
Cool-down after racing or workout,
        207, 226–27

Cooperating during race, 161–62
Cordain, Loren, <u>45</u>
Core and sprinting, <u>106</u>
Core strength training exercises
    effects of, 75
    Mountain Climbers, 75, **75**
    Plank with Alternating Knee Drops,
        76, **76**
    Prone Snow Angels, 75, **75**
    Seated Boat with Isometric Side
        Push, 76, **76**
Corneal abrasion, 238
Cornering
    apex of turn and, 102, 117, 193,
        197–98, 203
    arc of, carving smooth, 102
    braking and, 100–102
    countersteering and, 102
    crashing on hazardous, 116
    in criterium races, 165–66
    in cyclocross, 184
    while descending, 108
    drill, 193
    essentials, 101–2
    exiting, 102, 202–3
    leaning bike and, 102
    line changes and, 103
    in mountain bike races and riding,
        192–93
    no-hands riding and, 115
    while pack riding, 102
    pedaling and, 102
    Pro Tip, <u>103</u>
    while racing, 102–3
    on sharp turns (more than 90
        degrees), 102–3
    skills, tips for, 101–3, **101**, **102**, **103**
    on switchbacks, 202–4, **202**
    terrain and, 101
    on wet surfaces, 102, <u>103</u>
Countersteering, 102
Counting strategies for mental
        toughness, <u>166</u>
Cramping, muscle, 246–48
Crashing bike
    checklist for aftermath of, 119–20
    concussions from, 250
    while cornering, 116
    cycling insurance and, 120–21
    falling off bike and, 118–19
    in first race, xii
    from half-wheeling, 117–18
    inevitability of, 115–16
    from keeping head down, 116–17
    linear acceleration impact from, 250
    from overlapped wheels, 116
    from road hazards, 118

    rotational acceleration impact from,
        250
    from tense riding, 118
Crawford, Rick, <u>235</u>
Criterium "crit" races
    attacking in, 166
    cornering in, 165–66
    describing, 150–51
    finding, 165
    pack riding in, **164**, 165
    prizes and, 164
    selecting, 151
    sprinting in, 167–68
    term used in, key, 151
    training for, 165–68, <u>169</u>
    workouts for, 168, <u>169</u>
"Crit." *See* Criterium races
Crit sprints workouts, 168, <u>169</u>
Croasdale, Wayne, 190, 192–94
Crowder, Shawn, 118–19
Cummins, Jim, 128
Curcumin, 53, 246
Cutting-Edge Cycling, 225
Cycling computer, 19, 20
Cycling insurance, 120–21
Cycling skills. *See also specific skill*
    aerobic system and, 5–6
    anaerobic system and, 6–7
    braking, 100–102
    climbing, 108–11, **109**, **110**, **111**
    cornering, 101–3, **102**, **103**, 108
    descending, 107–8, **107**, <u>108</u>
    importance of, 99–100
    improving, 114–15, 144
    lactic acid and, 7–8
    limits and, pushing physical, 2, 8–9
    muscular system and, 4–5
    no-hands riding, 114–15
    one-hand riding, 114
    pacelining, 115, **115**
    pedaling, 103–5, **104**
    sprinting, 105, **105**, <u>106–7</u>
Cycling weight, ideal. *See also* Weight
    body shape and, <u>222</u>
    determining, 214–17, 215
    diet and, 220–21
    get leaner and faster, 215–16
    importance of, 213–14
    maintaining, 221–23
    power output and, 213
    power-to-weight ratio and, <u>221</u>
    reaching, plan for, 217–19
Cyclist's Training Bible, The, 46
Cyclocross
    appeal of, 178
    bike maintenance before racing,
        178–79

bike preparation for, 178–79
bikes for, <u>182</u>, <u>183</u>
bunny hop move in, 184
cornering in, 184
descending in, 183–84, <u>184</u>
describing, 151, 177, <u>180–81</u>
historical perspective of, 177
mountain bike for, <u>183</u>
obstacles in, handling, 179, 182–83
practicing course before racing, <u>178</u>
preparing for, 178–79
Pro Tip, <u>178</u>
selecting, 151
shouldering bike in, 182, **183**
term used in, key, 151–52
training for, 184–85, <u>186–87</u>
workouts for, 185, <u>186–87</u>
Cyclosportives. *See* Gran fondos

D

Dairy products, 48, 54, 253
Danielson, Tom, 75
Davenport, Paul, 33–34
Dead zone syndrome, avoiding, 31
Decaffeinated tea, 245–46
Deep breathing, 35
Dehydration, 61–62
Delayed-onset muscle soreness, 53, 245
Depression as overtraining symptom,
    232
Descending
    body position for, 108
    cornering while, 108
    in cyclocross, 183–84, <u>184</u>
    drill, 196
    in mountain bike races and riding,
        196–97, **196**
    pedaling while, <u>108</u>
    Pro Tip, <u>108</u>, <u>184</u>
    rules for, 108
    skills, tips for, 107–8, **107**, <u>108</u>
Dickson, Thomas, 83
Diet. *See also specific food*
    active rest and, 229
    breakfast and, <u>55</u>, 62–63, 223
    building blocks of, 42
    caffeine in, 60–62
    calcium in, 53–54
    carbohydrates in, 42–45, 47, <u>47</u>
    century rides and, 125–28
    cycling weight and, ideal, 220–21
    dietary fats in, 49–50, <u>50</u>, 52
    dinner and, 63
    energy bars and, 55–56, **55**
    glucose in, <u>45</u>
    gluten-free food in, <u>44</u>

glycemic index and, 47
herbs in, 52
improving, 50–55
in inflammation prevention, 53, <u>242</u>
in injury prevention, 252–54
iron in, <u>48</u>
lunch and, 63
meal replacement bars and, 57
Mediterranean, 50–52
metabolism and, 46, 221
one-hand riding while fueling and, 114
in pain management, 245–46
Paleo, 42, <u>45</u>
performance and, 41–42
postworkout, <u>64</u>
prerace, 62–64, 126–27
protein in, 47–48, 52
while racing, 64, <u>65</u>, 66, 207
racing and, 62–64, <u>65</u>, 66
recovery and, 229
recovery bars and, 56
snacks and, 62–63
spices in, 52
sugar in, 46–47
traumatic brain injury and, 252–54
vegetarian, <u>53</u>
vitamin D in, 54–55
weight loss and, body, 220–21
for women, <u>48</u>
women's bars and, 56–57
Dietary fats
    bad, 50
    body fat and, 49
    caffeine and, 60
    in diet, 49–50, <u>50</u>, 52
    good, 49
    importance of, 49
    intake of, recommended, 50, <u>50</u>
    monounsaturated, 49–50, 52
    muscles and, 49–50
    omega-3 fatty acids, 49–50, <u>50</u>, 53,
        246, 254
    plant-based, 52
    polyunsaturated, 49
    recommended daily intake of, 50
    saturated, 49
    sources of, <u>50</u>
    trans fats, 49
Dinner, 63
Dinowitz, Alyssa, 88
Double century rides, 128–29
Downhills. *See* Descending
Drafting, 141
Driller, Matt, 234
Drills. *See also* Training; Workouts
    attacking, 113
    braking, 195

climbing, 113, 191
cornering, 193
descending, 196
endurance, 113
obstacles, handling, 194
passing, 191
shifting, 192
sprinting, 112–13
trail reading, 195
Drinks. *See also* Hydration
    alcoholic, 220–21, 230–31
    caffeinated, 60–62
    carbohydrate, 45, 58
    electrolyte, 54, 220, 229
    energy, 207
    protein, 58
    recovery, <u>235</u>
    sports, 58, 60, 63–64, 66
    testing, 60
Drugs and sleep problems, 231
Dual x-ray absorptiometry (DXA)
    scan, 32
Duffield, Rob, 234, 236
Dugas, Jonathan, 4–6
Dumbbells, 81
DXA scan, 32
Dynamic stretching, 84

E

Eastern Fat Tire Association, 152
Ectomorph body shape, <u>222</u>
Efficiency and efficiency tests,
    35–37
Eggs, 48
Electrolyte drinks, 54, 220, 229
Eller, Mark, <u>198</u>
Emergency braking, 100–101
Endomorph body shape, <u>222</u>
Endurance
    caffeine and, 60
    carbohydrates and, 42–43
    drill, 113
    improving, 113
    training, 143
    training zone, 30, <u>30</u>
    workouts, 113, 135, <u>135</u>, 143, <u>144–45</u>,
        207, <u>208–9</u>
Energy, 6, 8
Energy bars, 55–56, **55**
Energy drinks, 207
Enzymes, 5–6, 13
Equipment. *See* Gear
Exercise
    explosive jumping, 77, <u>77</u>
    hydration during, 58

Exercise (*cont.*)
  intensity, 13–14, 24–25
  knee, 72, 243–44
  strength training
    abdominals, 80
    arms, 77–78, **78**
    back, 80
    during base period, 70–78, **70–78**
    during build period, 79–80
    core, 75–76, **75–76**
    glutes, 73–74, **73–74**
    knee, 72
    legs, 70–72, **70–72**, 79–80
    during peak period, 80–81
    shoulders, 81
    warm-up, 68–69, **68–69**
    wrists, 244–45
  stretching
    Baseboard Blast, 249
    Cat Cow, 88
    Chest Opener, 91, **91**
    Eagle Arm Pose, 88
    foam roller, 93–95, **93–95**
    Hip Flexor Stretch, 89, **89**
    Kneeling Lunge, 86, **86**
    Leg Roll, 85, **85**
    Lying Quad Stretch, 85, **85**
    Pigeon Pose, 86, **86**
    Shoulder Stand Scissors Kick,
      92, **92**
    Single Heel Drop Stand, 87, **87**
    Spinal Twist, 88
    Stair Drop, The, 249
    Standing Forward Fold, 87, **87**
    Straddle-Seated Windmill, 90, **90**
    Thigh Lengthener, 91, **91**
    Tilt and Hold, 88
    Wrist Stretch, 245
  talk test and, 13–14
  yoga-based
    back pain management and, 89
    Cat Cow, 88
    Eagle Arm Pose, 88
    Spinal Twist, 88
    Tilt and Hold, 88
Explosive jumping exercises, 77, 77
Eye injury, 238
Eyewear, 238

F

Falling off bike, 118–19. *See also*
    Crashing bike
Fartlek, 30
Fast-twitch muscle fiber, 4–5, 32–33
Fatigue, 90, 109, 232

Fat. *See* Body fat; Dietary fat
Feed zone, 150
Feedzone Cookbook, The, 28
Ferrentino, Mike, 131
Field House at Chelsea Piers, 119
Finger position and braking, 100
Fish, 49, 52, 246, 254
Fit, bike, 32, 139, 171–72
Fitness fundamentals. *See also* Lactic
    acid; Muscles
  aerobic system, 5–6
  anaerobic system, 6–7
  car analogy to human, 3
  lactic acid and, 7–8
  limits and, pushing physical, 4, 8–9
  muscles and muscular system, 4–5
  overview of, xiii
  perceived exertion rate and, 24–25
Flexibility. *See also* Stretching
  importance of, 83
  stretching and, 83
  tests for bicycling
    calves, 87, **87**
    glues, 86, **86**
    hamstrings, 87, **87**
    iliotibial band, quads, hip flexors,
      84–86, **84–86**
    touching toes and, 90
Foam roller stretching exercises
  back, 94, **94**
  calves, 95, **95**
  glutes, 93, **93**
  hamstrings, 93, **93**
  iliotibial band, 94, **94**
  quads, 94, **94**
Food. *See* Diet; *specific food*
Foot pain, 139, 244
Foot soreness, 139
Forks, setting and checking bike, 205
Frame, checking after crashing bike, 120
Frame size of body, 215, 215
Friel, Joe, 13, 45, 46, 217
Fries, Richard, 132
Frozen foods, 52
Fruits, 53, 246
Fund-raising goals, 133–34
Fürst, Silvia, 190–93, 195–96

G

Ganio, Matthew, 60–62
Gastrointestinal distress, 44
Gear. *See also* Bike
  carrying, while riding, 128
  for century rides, 129
  checking, 204

  clothing, 140, 233–34, **233**, 236
  for gran fondos, 140
  for home strength training, 81
  new, avoiding on race day, 155
  shoes, racing, 244
  stationary bike trainer, 24
  training, 19–20
Gear changes. *See* Shifting
Gidus, Tara, 55
Gilmartin, Shannon, 133–34, **133**
Gladden, Bruce L., 8
Glucose, 42, 44, 45
Gluten-free food, 44
Gluten sensitivity, 44
Glutes
  bicycling flexibility test, 86, **86**
  foam roller stretching exercise, 93, **93**
  strength training exercises
    Clam, 74, **74**
    effects of, 73
    importance of, 73
    Side Step, 74, **74**
    Single-Leg Bridge, 73, **73**
  stretching, 86, **86**
Glycemic index, 47
Glycogen, 5, 8, 56, 220
Go to Bicycling.com, 142
GPS-enabled computer, 20
Grains, 48
Gran fondos
  century rides vs., 138, 138
  clothing for, 140
  describing, 138
  drafting in, 141
  finding, 142
  gear for, 140
  mass start and, 141
  pacing in, 141–42
  planning for, 140
  prerace preparation for, 142
  Pro Tip, 143
  race day preparation for, 142–43
  starting, 141, 141
  term of, 139
  tips for, 139–43, 141, 143
  training for, 143–44, 144–45
  workouts for, 143–44, 144–45
Green tea, 245
Grouchiness as overtraining symptom,
  232
Group ride workouts, 143, 162, 168. *See*
  also Pack riding
Guerra, Jeff, 243
Guzman, Anne, 220
Gymnastics class for practicing falling,
  119

H

Hair follicle, inflamed or ingrown, 238, 240
Haldeman, Lon, 67
Half-wheeling, avoiding, 117–18
Hall, Gina, 183–85
Hamstrings
　bicycling flexibility test, 87, **87**
　foam roller stretching exercise, 93, **93**
　strain, 248
　strength training exercise, 82
　stretching, 87, **87**
Handlebars, 171–72
Hand pain, 244–45, 245
Hand position, changing, 245
Hand-ups, 151–52
Harr, Eric, 34–35
Head position, avoiding keeping down, 116–17
Heart and aerobic capacity, 5–6
Heart disease, 46, 90
Heart palpitations as overtraining symptom, 231–32
Heart rate
　factors affecting, 27
　maximum, 6–7, 23, 25
　monitoring, 20, 22, 27, 31
　racing, 231–32
　resting, 19, 231
　tests, 21–23
　training and, 21–23
　zones, 21–22
Heart rate monitor, 20, 22, 27, 31
Helmet, bike, 119–20, 250
Helping another biker while riding, 114
Henderson, Neal, 15–16, 29, 31
Herbs, 52
Herrera, James, 28, 162
Hill accelerations workouts, 110–11, 207, 208–9
Hillard, Tom, 190–96
Hills. *See also* Climbing; Descending
　long, steady, 109
　rolling, 109–10
　short, steep, 110
　training for, 109–11, 143
Hill sprints workouts, 111, 185, 186–87, 207, 208–9
Hinton, Pamela, 32
Hip flexors
　bicycling flexibility test, 84–86, **84–86**
　stretching, 84–86, **84–86**, 89, **89**
Hollis, Bruce, 54–55
Holz, Scott, 83–84, 172
Home lactate threshold test, 26–27

Home strength training equipment and gear, 81
Home strength training exercises, 82
Horner, Chris, 135, 225
Hot weather and hydration, 59–60
Hydration
　black mold in water bottle and, 240
　caffeinated drinks, 60–62
　caffeine and, 61
　carbohydrate drinks, 45, 58
　century rides and, 125, 127
　cramping and, preventing, 247
　daily, 58–59
　electrolyte drinks, 54, 220, 229
　during exercise, 58
　facts about, 57–59
　guidelines, 66
　in hot weather, 59–60
　one-hand riding and, 114
　performance and, 59
　perspiration and, 57
　prerace, 57–58, 59
　protein drinks, 58
　during race, 66
　recovery drink, 235
　replacing lost fluid and, 57
　sports drinks, 60, 63–64, 66
　testing drinks and, 60
　water, 59–60

I

Iannetta, Sam, 70
Ibuprofen, 53, 245
Iglinsky, Maxim, 116
Iliotibial band
　bicycling flexibility test, 84–86, **84–86**
　foam roller stretching exercise, 94, **94**
　friction syndrome, 85
　stretching exercises, 84–86, **84–86**
Inclines. *See* Climbing; Descending; Hills
Individuality of training, 12
Infected road rash, 239–40
Inflammation
　of hair follicle, 238
　insulin and, 46
　preventing and treating
　　berries, 53
　　diet, 53, 242
　　ibuprofen, 53
　　omega-3 fatty acids and, 49, 53
　　recovery, 227
　　RICE treatment, 242
　sugar and, 46
　training and, 4

Ingrown hair follicle, 240
Injuries. *See also* Pain and pain management
　brain, 249–54
　chafing, 240–41
　corneal abrasion, 238
　diet in preventing, 252–54
　hair follicle, inflamed or ingrown, 238, 240
　occurrences of, 237
　overuse, 88
　overview of, xiii
　road rash, 239–40, 240
　saddle sores, 238–39
　shoulder, 249
　wound care, 158
　wrist, 244–45
Insulin, 43, 46, 49
Insurance, cycling, 120–21
Intensity of exercise, 13–14, 24–25
International Society of sports Nutrition, 58
Iron, 48

J

Jefferson, Martha, 230
Jeukendrup, Asker, 43–45
Johnson, Tim, 114–15, 116–19, 141–42, 143, 178
Jump phase of sprint, 106, 107

K

Kadlick, Margaret, 6
Kaelin, Darryl, 251–52
Karpets, Vladimir, 116
Kelinson, Adam, 54
Knees
　exercise, 72, 243–44
　pain in, 243–44
　warmers, removing while riding, 114
　wobbling of, avoiding, 103
Kropelnicki, Jesse, 231
Kyle, Chester, 158

L

Lactate. *See* Lactic acid
Lactate threshold. *See also* Lactic acid
　defining, 6
　determining, 25–27, 32
　intervals workout, with bursts, 185, 186–87
　power and, riding at sustained high level of, 14, 170

Lactate threshold (*cont.*)
  tests, 25–27, <u>32</u>
  training and
    as baseline measurement, 30, <u>30</u>
    intensity and, 24–25
    misnomer of, 7
    training zone, 30, <u>30</u>
Lactic acid. *See also* Lactate threshold
  acidosis and, 7
  cool-downs and, 227
  cycling skills and, 7–8
  energy and, 8
  minutes needed to clear after
    exercise, <u>7</u>
  muscles and, 7–8
  production of, 6–8
  theory of, disputed, 7
  training and, 7–8
Lange, Hank, 24
LDL cholesterol, 50
Leader's jersey, 151
Legal waivers, 153–54, <u>153</u>
Leg strength training exercises
  Bulgarian Squat, 70, **70**
  Double Leg Curl, 82
  Dumbbell Squat to Overhead Press,
    71, **71**
  Dumbbell T, 82
  effects of, 70
  Hamstring Stretch, 82
  High Step, 79
  Jack Squats, 79
  Lunge Jumps, 79–80
  Single-Leg Step Down, 71, **71**
  Slider Squat, 71, **71**
  Sliding Lunge, 82
  Stability Ball Hamstring Curl, 72, **72**
  Step-Up, 82
  weights for, 70
LeMond, Greg, 104
Levin, Scott, 93
Lewin, Barbara, 245–46
Lewis, Craig, 118–19, 233
Lewis, C. S., 99
Lim, Allen, 28, <u>44</u>
Limits, pushing physical, 2, 8–9
Linear acceleration impact from
    crashing bike, 250
Line changes and cornering, 103
Lockhart, Fiona, 249
Log, training, 19
Looking backward while racing, 161
Lumbar muscles strength training
    exercise, 80
Lunch, 63
Lungs and lung tests, 33–35

M

McCalvin, Reed, 227
McCormack, Mark, 28
McCrann, Patrick, 242
McHugh, Malachy, 84
Macrocycles
  base period of
    describing, 12–13
    sample year training, 16–17
    strength training during, 70–77,
      70–77
  build period of
    describing, 13
    sample year training, 17–18
    strength training during, 79–80
  defining, 12
  peak period of
    describing, 14
    sample year training, 18–19
    strength training during, 80–81
  sample year of training, 16–19
Magnesium, 247
Mah, Cherie, 230
Marlor, Donna, 43, <u>44</u>, 45
Martin, Jim, 172
Massage, 158, 227–28
Mass starts, tips for, <u>141</u>
Matheny, Fred, 21
Maximum heart rate, 6–7, 23, 25
Maximum VO$_2$
  builders workouts, 162, <u>163</u>
  of cyclists, elite, 6
  during endurance drill, 113
  improving, 6, 23
  intervals workouts, 162, <u>163</u>, 168, <u>169</u>,
    207, <u>208–9</u>
  perceived exertion studies and, 23
  training zone, 30, <u>30</u>
Meal replacement bars, 57
Meat, lean, 253
Medications and sleep problems,
    231
Mediterranean diet, 50–52
Melatonin production, 230–31
Mental toughness, <u>166</u>
Merckx, Eddy, 31, 213
Mesomorph body shape, <u>222</u>
Metabolism, 46, 221
Meyerhof, Otto, 7
Micro bursts workouts, 185, <u>186–87</u>
Microcycles, 15–18
Miles, Mary, 245
Milk, 48
Milk protein, 49
Millard-Stafford, Mindy, 61

Miller, Meredith, 115
Minerals. *See specific type*
Mionskie, Bob, 120
Miserableness as overtraining
    symptom, 232
Mitochondria, 5, 7, 13
Monounsaturated fats, 49–50, 52
Moore, Greg, 67
Morgan, Molly, 61
Mountain bike races and riding
  bike for, <u>183</u>
  braking in, 195–96
  breakdowns and, preparing for, 204,
    <u>205</u>, 206
  climbing in, 191–92
  cool-down after, 207
  cornering in, 192–93
  descending in, 196–97, **196**
  describing, 151
  first, surviving, 204, 206–7
  obstacles in, handling, 193–94,
    194
  pacing in, 206
  passing in, 191, <u>198</u>
  personal experience of, 189–90
  railing a berm in, 197–98
  refueling during, 207
  roll-through move in, 199
  selecting, 151
  shifting in, 192
  shouldering bike in, 199
  suspension and, setting and
    checking, <u>205</u>
  switchbacks in, 202–4, **202**
  term used in, key, 151
  trail etiquette and, <u>198</u>
  trail reading in, 195
  training for, 207, <u>208–9</u>
  V-dip in, 198–200
  warm-up before, 206
  waterways in, navigating, 200–202,
    201
  wet surfaces and, <u>200</u>
  wheelie move in, 199–200
  workouts for, 207, <u>208–9</u>
Muhich, Lisa, 177
Mulholland, Owen, 159
Muscles. *See also specific type*
  acid generated by, 6
  adaptation and, 226
  burning in, 8
  caffeine and, 60
  carbohydrates and, 8
  cramping, 246–48
  cycling skills and, 4–5
  dietary fats and, 49–50

fiber types
    fast-twitch, 4–5, 32–33
    power output and, 5
    slow-twitch, 4–5, 32–33
    tests, 32–33
    fitness fundamentals and, 4–5
glycogen and, tapping of, 5, 8
lactic acid and, 7–8
lean mass, 47, 74
massage and, 227
postexercise, 63
protein and, 47, 63, 74
soreness of, 8, 53, 245
sugar and, 46
training and, 226
Myerson, Adam, 179, 180–81, 182–83

N

Napping, 231
National Electronic Injury Surveillance
    System, 250
National Weight Control Registry, 222
Neel, Mike, 11
Neuromuscular power training zone,
    30, 31
Newtown, Harvey, 32
Niles, Rick, 25
Nissila, Juuso, 35
No-hands riding, 114–15
Nonsteroidal anti-inflammatory drugs,
    245
"No pain/no gain" philosophy of
    training, 23
Number, pinning on race, 155–56, **156**
Nutrition. *See* Diet; *specific food*

O

Obstacles, handling
    in cyclocross, 179, 182–83
    drill, 194
    in mountain bike races and riding,
        193–94, **194**
Omega-3 fatty acids, 49–50, 50, 53,
    246, 254
One-day road races
    attacking in, 161
    breaking away in, 161–62
    describing, 150
    postrace preparation for, 161
    prerace preparation for, 160
    race day preparation for, 160–61
    selecting, 150
    term used in, key, 150
    training for, 162, 163
    workouts for, 162, 163

One-hand riding, 114
On-the-bike lung test, 34
Oregon Bicycle Racing Association, 152
Osguthorpe, Jeff, 190, 193
Overend, Ned, 123, 149, 190–92, 194,
    196, 204
Overexertion, avoiding, 248
Overlapped wheels, avoiding, 116
Overload, 12, 27
Overton, Frank, 165–66
Overtraining, avoiding, 25, 28, 231–33
Over unders workout, 111
Overuse injuries, 88
Oxidative stress, 245
Oxygen, 5–6

P

Pacelining, 115–16, **115**
Pacing
    in century rides, 125
    in gran fondos, 141–42
    in mountain bike races, 206
    sprints, 106
Pack riding
    anxiety about, 114
    in charity rides, 134, 135
    climbing while, 110
    cornering and, 102
    in criterium races, **164**, 165
    Pro Tip, 135
Pack-Riding Anxiety Disorder, 114
Pain and pain management. *See also*
    Injuries
    Achilles tendinitis, 248–49
    back, 88, 89
    collarbone fractures, 249
    concussions, 249–54
    cramping, 246–48
    delayed-onset muscle soreness, 53,
        245
    diet and, 245–46
    foot, 139, 244
    hamstring strain, 248
    hand, 244–45, 245
    iliotibial band friction syndrome, 85
    knees, 243–44
    muscle soreness, 8, 53, 245
    nonsteroidal anti-inflammatory
        drugs and, 245
    preventative strategies, 245–46
    shoulder, 249
    tea and, 245–46
    traumatic brain injury, 249–54
    ulnar nerve, 244
    upper body, 242–43

Paleo diet, 42, 45
Paleo Diet for Athletes, The, 46
Parathyroid hormone, 54
Parker, Tim, 237
Park, Peter, 68
Passing
    drill, 191
    in mountain bike races and riding,
        191, 198
Peak period of macrocycle
    describing, 14
    sample year training, 18–19
    strength training during, 80–81
Pedaling
    climbing and, 110
    cornering and, 102
    while descending, 108
    hip-knee-angle alignment and,
        103–5
    knee wobble and, avoiding, 103
    LeMond's advice on, 104
    power phase of, 103–4
    saddle position and, 105
    shifting and, 104
    skills, tips ford, 103–5, **104**
    on switchbacks, 203
Pedal stroke analysis, 32
Pedal strokes, counting, 166
Peiffer, Jeremiah, 234
Pelotonaphobia, 114
Perceived exertion rate and tests,
    22–25, 31, 218
Performance
    caffeine and, 60–62
    calcium and, 54
    carbohydrates and, 45
    diet and, 41–42
    hydration and, 59
    improvement in, 11
    plateau, 12
    power-to-weight ratio and, 221
    sleep and, 230
    training and, 62
    vitamin D and, 54
    warm-up and, 157
    weight loss and, 220
Periodization, 12, 15–16
Perspiration, 57, 59
Phillips, Stuart, 73, 74
Physiological tests
    bicycling flexibility, 84–87, **84–87**
    bike fit, dynamic, 32
    bone density, 32
    efficiency, 35–37
    heart rate, 21–23
    lactate threshold, 25–27, 32

Physiological tests (*cont.*)
lungs, 33–35
muscle type, 32–33
perceived exertion rate, 22–25
power output, 28–29, 29
Plyo box or step, 81
Plyometric training, 77, 77, 222
Polyunsaturated fats, 49
Postcrash checklist, 119–20
Postworkout diet, 64
Potassium, 52–53, 229
Power
defining, 5
developing, 5
intervals workouts, 207, 208–9
lactate threshold and riding at
sustained high level of, 14, 170
output
caffeine and, 60
cycling weight and, ideal, 213
importance of, 21
measuring, 20, 22, 27
muscle fibers and, 5
professional vs. recreational
riders, 29, 29
tests, 28–29, 29
training and, 21–22
wattage, generating, 27–28, 29
pedaling phase, 103–4
tests, 28–29, 29
threshold, 28, 170
training for, 5
weight and, body, 213
Power meter, 20, 22, 27–28
Powers, Jeremy, 183
Power-to-weight ratio, 221
Prerace diet, 62–64, 126–27
Price, Daryl, 204
Prime (prize), 151, 164
Prizes, racing, 151, 164
Processed food, 43
Progression, training, 12
Protein
absorption of, 48–49
bars, 56
in diet, 47–48, 52
drinks, 58
function of, 47
glycemic index and, 57
importance of, 47–48
intake of, recommended, 47–48
lean muscle mass and, 47, 74
muscles and, 47, 63, 74
shake, 229
sources of, 48–49, 63, 63
in sports drinks, 58

swapping sources of, 52
in wheat, 44
Pro Tip
breathing, 133
climbing, 110, 111
cornering, 103
cyclocross, 178
descending, 108, 184
gear, avoiding new on race day, 155
gran fondos, 143
hand position, changing, 245
jump phase of sprint, 107
lactate threshold test, 32
pack riding in charity rides, 135
practice laps before cyclocross, 178
rest on day before racing, avoiding,
154
shifting, 104, 125
training goals, 15
unplugging from heart rate monitor,
31
wet riding surfaces, 171, 200
Pruitt, Andrew "Andy," 84

Q
Quads
bicycling flexibility text, 84–86,
84–86
foam roller stretching exercise, 94,
94
stretching, 84–86, **84–86**
Quinoa, 48

R
Race number, pinning on, 155–56, **156**
Racing. *See also specific race*
breaking away while, 161–62
cool-down after, 207
cooperating while, 161–62
cornering while, 102–3
diet and, 62–64, 65, 66
diet while, 64, 65, 66, 207
feeling of, 149
finding race nearby, 152
increase in participants in, xii-xiii
key terms, 150–52
looking backward and, 161
mental toughness and, 166
options, 131–32
overview of, xiii
personal experience with first, xi-xii
preparing for, 154–55, 154, 155
prizes, 151, 164
registering for race, 152

rest on day before, avoiding, 155
safety tips, 160
shaving legs and, 155
speed vs. smoothness, 171
style tips for, 155–57
terms, key, 150–52
urination during, 156
waivers for, legal, 153–54, 153
warm-up before, 157, 157, 206
winning race and, 150
Railing a berm, 197–98
Rainy conditions, 102, 103, 171, 200
Rear derailleur and cranks, checking
after crashing, 120
Rebound, measuring bike suspension's,
205
Recovery
active
training zone, 30, 30
workouts, 135, 135, 143, 144–45,
207, 208–9
bars, 56
cold bath and, 228–29, **228**
compression clothing and, 233–34,
233, 236
diet and, 229
drink, 235
importance of, 225–26
inflammation and, avoiding, 227
massage and, 227–28
need for, 226, 226
overload and, 12, 27
overtraining and, avoiding, 231–33
rest and, active, 226–31
sleep and, 230–31
Refined food, 43
Registering for race, 152
Resistance bands, 81
Rest. *See also Recovery*
active
cold bath, 228–29, **228**
cool-down after workout, 226–27
diet and, 229
massage, 227–28
sleep and, 230–31
during century rides, 125, 127
on day before race, avoiding, 154
importance of, 14–15
Pro Tip, 154
as training component, 14–15
Resting heart rate, 19, 231
Rey, Hans, 114
Rice, 48
RICE (rest, ice, compression, elevation)
treatment, 242
"Right rear" rule, 100

Rims, cleaning bike, 178
"Ring" technique, 115
Road bike, 182
Road hazards, avoiding, 118
Road races. *See* Racing; *specific race*
Road rash, 239–40, 240
Road skills. *See* Cycling skills
Roll-through move, 199
Rominger, Tony, 41
Ross, Brad, 178
Rotational acceleration impact from
     crashing bike, 250
Rusch, Rebecca, 189
Russ, Matt, 32
Rutledge, Tim, 178
Ryan, Monique, 57–59, 126–27, 142

S

Saddle
    Achilles tendinitis and, 248–49
    angle, 172
    fitting, 241
    hamstring strain and, 248
    height, 172
    position, 105, 171
    sores, 238–39
Safety tips
    racing, 160
    wet riding surfaces, 102, 103, 171, 200
Sag, measuring bike suspension's, 205
Salmon, 246
Salt, 53–54, 229, 247
Saltonstall, Anna, 248
San Millán, Iñigo, 41–42, 64
Sass, Cynthia, 51–52, 55–56, 242, 252–54
Saturated fats, 49
Saxena, Amol, 244
Scherb, Cliff, 14–15
Science of Sport, The, blog, 4
Seafood, 49, 52, 246, 254
Seasonings, food, 52
Seatpost, 171–72
Separated shoulder, 249
Shaving legs for racing, 158
Shea, Marti, 139
Shelby, Dan, 8–9
Shifting
    cadence and, 125
    while climbing, 111, 139
    drill, 192
    in moutain bike races and riding, 192
    pedaling and, 104
    Pro Tip, 104, 125
    smooth, 104, 125
    on switchbacks, 202

Shocks, setting and adjusting bike,
     205
Shoes, fitting, 244
Shoes, racing, 244
Shouldering bike, 182, **183**, 199
Shoulders
    injuries to, 249
    pain in, 249
    strength training exercise, 81
Simple carbohydrates, 43
Sims, Stacy T., 43, 44, 45, 45, 60
Singletrack, 151
Skateboarding for practicing falling, 119
Skin injuries
    chafing, 240–41
    hair follicle, inflamed or ingrown,
         238, 240
    road rash, 239–40, 240
    saddle sores, 238–39
Slacking, preventing, 28
Sleep, 19, 229–31
Sliding discs, 81
Slow-twitch muscle fiber, 4–5, 32–33
Smith, Douglas H., 252
Smoothness vs. speed, racing, 171
Snacks, 62–63
Socks, choosing, 244
Sodium, 53–54, 229, 247
Soybeans, 246
Soy milk, 246
Soy nuts, 246
Specialized's Body Geometry Saddle
     Fit System, 241
Specificity of training, 12
Speed play, 30
Speed vs. smoothness, racing, 171
Spices, 52
Spin, sharpening, 28
Sports drinks, 58, 60, 63–64, 66
Sports Nutrition for Endurance Athletes,
     57, 142
Sprinting
    body position and, 106
    core and, 106
    in criterium races, 167–68
    drill, 112–13
    improving, 112–13
    natural vs. learned, 106
    pacing, 106
    phases of, 106, 107
    questions about, 106–7
    skills, tips for, 105, **105**, 106–7
    winning, tips for, 167
    wobbling during, 107
    workouts, 112–13
Squish test for shoe fit, 244

SST crisscross intervals workouts, 185,
     186–87
SST interval workouts, 168, **169**, 173,
     174–75
Stabile, Jon, 240
Stability ball, 81
Stage races, 151
Start intervals workouts, 173, 174–75
Static stretching, 84
Stationary bike trainer, 24
Stationary trainer, power-enabled, 28
Steady state workouts, 207, 208–9
Steak, 74
Steering area, checking after crashing,
     120
Stern, Richard, 16
Stevens, Evelyn "Evie," 99–100
Stewart, Jeb, 112–13
Stopping. *See* Braking
Strength training
    abdominals, 80
    arms
        Applause Pushup, 80
        effects of, 77
        Hammer Curl, 78, **78**
        Lying Triceps Extension, 78, **78**
        Military Pushup, 78, **78**
    back, 80
    during base period, 70–78, **70–78**
    beef and, eating before, 74
    during build period, 79–80
    core
        effects of, 75
        Mountain Climbers, 75, **75**
        Plank with Alternating Knee
            Drops, 76, **76**
        Prone Snow Angels, 75, **75**
        Seated Boat with Isometric Side
            Push, 76, **76**
    glutes
        Clam, 74, **74**
        effects of, 73
        importance of, 73
        Side Step, 74, **74**
        Single-Leg Bridge, 73, **73**
    hamstrings, 82
    at home, 81–82
    importance of, 67
    knee extensors, 72
    lean muscle mass and, 74
    legs
        Bulgarian Squat, 70, **70**
        Double Leg Curl, 82
        Dumbbell Squat to Overhead
            Press, 71, **71**
        Dumbbell T, 82

Strength training (*cont.*)
  legs (*cont.*)
    effects of, 70
    Hamstring Stretch, 82
    High Step, 79
    Jack Squats, 79
    Lunge Jumps, 79
    Single-Leg Step Down, 71, **71**
    Slider Squat, 71, **71**
    Sliding Lunge, 82
    Stability Ball Hamstring Curl,
      72, **72**
    Step-Up, 82
    weights for, 70
  lumbar muscles, 80
  during peak period, 80–81
  plyometric training, 77, **77**
  sedentary work style and, 68
  shoulders, 81
  trapezius, 81
  warm-up
    Founder, The, 68, **68**
    importance of, 68
    Lunge Stretch, The, 69, **69**
    Wall Squat, The, 69, **69**
  weights for, 70, 73, 79
  wrists, 244–45
Strength Training for Cyclists videos, 32
Stress management and breathing, 133
Stretching. *See also* Flexibility
  back, 88
  calves, 87, **87**
  consistency and, 84
  dynamic, 84
  exercises
    Baseboard Blast, 249
    Cat Cow, 88
    Chest Opener, 91, **91**
    Eagle Arm Pose, 88
    foam roller, 93–95, **93–95**
    Hip Flexor Stretch, 89, **89**
    Kneeling Lunge, 86, **86**
    Leg Roll, 85, **85**
    Lying Quad Stretch, 85, **85**
    Pigeon Pose, 86, **86**
    Shoulder Stand Scissors Kick,
      92, **92**
    Single Heel Drop Stand, 87, **87**
    Spinal Twist, 88
    Stair Drop, The, 249
    Standing Forward Fold, 87, **87**
    Straddle-Seated Windmill,
      90, **90**
    Thigh Lengthener, 91, **91**
    Tilt and Hold, 88
    Wrist Stretch, 245

  flexibility and, 83
  glutes, 86, **86**
  hamstrings, 87, **87**
  hip flexors, 84–86, **84–86**, 89, **89**
  iliotibial band, 84–86, **84–86**
  importance of, 83
  in preventing
    Achilles tendinitis, 249
    cramping, 248
    fatigue, 90
  quads, 84–86, **84–86**
  static, 84
  timing of, 84
Style tips for racing, 155–57
Sugar, 46–47
Sunlight, exposure to, 54
Supplement, vitamin D, 55
Suspension, setting and checking,
    205
Swain, David, PhD, 15
Sweating, 57, 59
Sweeteners, 43
"Sweet spot," 30, 168, 173, 185
Swenson, Peter, 190, 192, 195–97
Switchbacks, handling, 202–4, **202**

T

Talk test, 13–14
Tanner, Todd, 190, 196–97
Tea, 245–46
Technique work, 144, 144–45
Tempo training zone, 30, 30
Tempo workouts, 144, 144–45, 207,
    208–9
Tense riding, avoiding, 118
Testa, Max, 4, 226–29, 227
Testosterone, 50
30/30/30/30 workouts, 185, 186–87
30-minute time trial, 26
Tilford, Steve, 190–91, 197
Time trial field test, 19, 22–23
Time trial races
  describing, 150, 170
  selecting, 150
  term used in, key, 150
  tips for, 170–72
  training for, 173, 174–75
  workouts for, 173, 174–75
Tire debris, clearing while riding,
    114
Tires, inflating, 179
Tofu, 246
Tomac, John, 189, 204, 206
Top end of sprint, 106
Touching toes and flexibility, 90

Trail etiquette, 198
Trail reading, 195
Training. *See also* Drills; Strength
      training; Workouts
  blended periodization, 15–16
  caffeine and, 61–62
  for carbohydrate intake, 45
  for century rides, 126, 128–29, 130
  for charity rides, 134–36, 135, 136–37
  for criterium races, 165–68, 169
  for cyclocross, 184–85, 186–87
  for double century rides, 128
  endurance, 143
  gear, 19–20
  goals, 15
  for gran fondos, 143–44, 144–45
  heart rate and, 21–23
  for hills, 109–11, 143
  individuality of, 12
  inflammation and, 4
  lactate threshold and
    as baseline measurement, 30, 30
    intensity and, 24–25
    misnomer of, 7
  lactic acid and, 7–8
  log, 19
  macrocycles
    base period, 12–13, 16–17
    build period, 13, 17–18
    defining, 12
    peak period, 14, 18–19
    sample year of, 16–19
  microcycle, 15–18
  for mountain bike races, 207, 208–9
  muscles and, 226
  "no pain/no gain" philosophy of, 23
  for one-day road race, 162, 163
  overload and, 12
  overview of, xiii
  performance and, 62
  periodization, 12, 15–16
  plyometric, 77, 77, 222
  for power, 5
  power output and, 21–22
  principles, 12
  progression, 12
  rest as component of, 14–15
  sample year
    base period of macrocycle, 16–17
    build period of macrocycle, 17–18
    peak period of macrocycle, 18–19
  specificity of, 12
  time trial field test and, 19, 22–23
  for time trial races, 173, 174–75
  web-based platform, 19
  zones, 22, 29–31, 30

Training and Racing with a Power Meter, 27
Train to Live, Live to Train, 242
Trans fats, 49
Trapezius strength training exercise, 81
Traumatic brain injury, 249–54
Trebon, Ryan, 240
Trexler, Lance, 252
Triathlon Training in Four Hours a Week, 34
Tuna, 246
Turmeric, 53, 246
Turning. *See* Cornering
20/20 crit sprints workouts, 168, **169**

U

Udani, Jay, 246
Ulnar nerve pain, 244
Union Cycliste Internationale, 236
Uphills. *See* Climbing
Upper body pain, 242–43
Urinating during race, 156
USA Cycling, xii-xiii, 131, 152, 159

V

V-dip move, 198–200
Vegetables, 52, 253
Vegetarian diet, 53
Velodrome, 118
Vertical jump test, 32–33
Victory salute move, 114–15
Vitamin C, 253
Vitamin D, 54–55, 253
Vitamin D deficiency, 55
Vitamins, 50. *See also specific type*

W

Waivers, legal, 153–54, 153
Warm-up before racing, 157, 157, 206
Warm-up exercises
  Founder, The, 68, **68**
  importance of, 68
  Lunge Stretch, The, 69, **69**
  Wall Squat, The, 69, **69**
Water intake, 59–60. *See also* Hydration
Waterways, navigating, 200–202, **201**

Wattage, generating power, 27–28, 29
Weak spots, pinpointing, 28
Weight, body. *See also* Cycling weight, ideal
  baseline for healthy, finding, 214
  loss, 49, 52, 214–15, 220–21
  power and, 213
  recording, 19, 223
Weights for strength training, 70, 73, 79
Westfahl, Allison, 75
Wet riding surfaces, 102, 103, 171, 200
Wheat and wheat allergies, 44
Wheat-free food, 44
Wheelie move, 199–200
Wheels
  avoiding overlapped, 116
  crashing bike and, checking after, 120
  rims of, cleaning, 178
Whey, 49
Wind, managing, 150, 170–71
Winter, Christopher, 230
Wobbling during sprinting, 107
Wobbling knees, avoiding, 103
Women's bars and diet, 48, 56–57
Workouts. *See also* Drills; Training
  active recovery, 135, 135, 143, 144–45, 207, 208–9
  anaerobic capacity power builders, 185, 186–87
  attacking, 113
  bike lifts, 185, 186–87
  brick, 185, 186–87
  bursts, 162, **163**, 173, 174–75, 185, 186–87
  for century rides, 129, 130
  for charity rides, 135–36, 135, 136–37
  climbing, 110–11, 113, 207, 208–9
  climb repeats, 207, 208–9
  cool-down after, 207, 226–27
  for criterium races, 168, 169
  crit sprints, 168, 169
  for cyclocross, 185, 186–87
  diet after, 64
  endurance, 113, 135, 135, 143, 144–45, 207, 208–9
  for gran fondos, 143–44, 144–45
  group ride, 143, 162, 168
  hill accelerations, 110–11, 207, 208–9

  hill sprints, 111, 185, 186–87, 207, 208–9
  hill work, 143, 144–45
  lactate threshold intervals with bursts, 185, 186–87
  maximum VO$_2$ builders, 162, 163
  maximum VO$_2$ intervals, 162, 163, 168, 169, 207, 208–9
  micro bursts, 185, 186–87
  for mountain bike races, 207, 208–9
  for one-day races, 162, 163
  over unders, 111
  power intervals, 207, 208–9
  sprinting, 112–13
  SST crisscross intervals, 185, 186–87
  SST intervals, 168, 169, 173, 174–75
  start intervals, 173, 174–75
  steady state, 207, 208–9
  technique, 144, 144–45
  tempo, 144, 144–45, 207, 208–9
  30/30/30/30, 185, 186–87
  for time trial races, 173, 174–75
  20/20 crit sprints, 168, 169
Wounds
  caring for, 158
  hair follicle, inflamed or ingrown, 238, 240
  road rash, 40, 239–40
  saddle sores, 238–39
  unhealed, 232
Wrist injuries and prevention, 244–45

Y

Yates, Sean, 114
Yoga-based exercises
  back pain management and, 88, 89
  Cat Cow, 88
  Eagle Arm Pose, 88
  Spinal Twist, 88
  Tilt and Hold, 88
Young, Roger, 116–17, 225

Z

Zabriskie, Dave, 172
Zeising, Hunter, 141
Zinc, 253–54

About the Editor

DANIELLE KOSECKI IS THE HEALTH EDITOR AT *GLAMOUR* MAGAZINE, where road rash is never on trend. A lifelong athlete, she discovered bike racing while dabbling in triathlon after her collegiate soccer career and never looked back. Kosecki is currently a category 2–road bike racer for CityMD Women's Racing Team but tackles the track and trails whenever possible. She lives in Brooklyn with her dreamy husband, two awesome cats, and not nearly enough bikes.